My Sweet Life

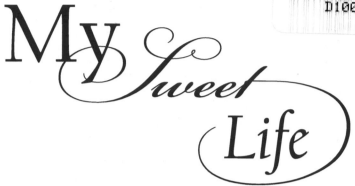

Successful Women with Diabetes

BEVERLY S. ADLER, PhD, CDE

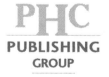
and Friends

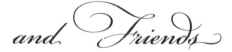

PHC
PUBLISHING
GROUP

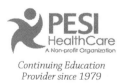
PESI
HealthCare
A Non-profit Organization
Continuing Education
Provider since 1979

PHC Publishing Group is an imprint of PESI HealthCare

Eau Claire, Wisconsin © 2011

For information on this book and other continuing education
materials from **PHC Publishing Group** or **PESI HealthCare**
please call **800-843-7763**
or visit our websites
www.phcpublishing.com
www.pesihealthcare.com

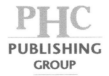 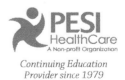

PHC Publishing Group is an imprint of PESI HealthCare

Cover art by Jan A. Sullivan | www.retroartbyjan.com

A portion of the proceeds from the sale of this book will be donated, on behalf of the author and the contributing writers, to the American Diabetes Association.

Acknowledgements

First, and foremost, I would like to express my deepest gratitude to the twenty-three successful women with diabetes who joined me in sharing their inspiring life stories. Although they make living a successful life look easy, it surely is not. With their contributions to this book, we do not have to re-invent the wheel – by which I mean, we can benefit from their insight and the lessons they've learned as they manage their diabetes along with career and/or family. Thank you, my "diabetes sisters!"

I would like to thank Heidi Strosahl Knower, my publisher at PHC Publishing Group, for bringing my dream to print. She encouraged my ideas, respected my choices, and matched my enthusiasm with her own, for this project. Thanks also to Barb Caffrey and Yvonne Kuter for their editorial contributions.

I would like to express my heartfelt gratitude to my peer reviewer, Susan Weiner, RD, MS, CDE, CDN, Registered Dietitian and Certified Diabetes Educator, for her insightful comments. Despite her full schedule, she managed to devote time to reviewing the chapters. I'm so happy I could rely on her extensive knowledge about nutrition to ensure accurate nutritional information.

I would like to thank my friend, Jeanne Dippel, for her help managing the authors' photos. Her assistance was greatly appreciated.

I would like to thank my sweet suite partner, Alfred Lewis, LCSW, for his wit and wisdom throughout this process.

I would like to thank my mother, my sister, Evelyn, and my sister-in-law, Ella, for their continued moral support.

Last, but not least, I want to express my love and thanks to my wonderful children, Harrison and Taylor. I am totally indebted to them for providing me with technological expertise (Harrison) and fashion expertise (Taylor). I am blessed to have their loving support as I pursue my goals.

Beverly S. Adler, PhD, CDE

Dedication

This book is dedicated, in loving memory, to the three most important men who have graced my life: my father, Dr. Helmut E. Adler (1920-2001), my brother, Barry Peter Adler (1945-2009), and my beloved soul mate, Dr. Daniel Bruno (1954-2007). Each man supported my dreams, encouraged my goals, and shared in the joy of my accomplishments. They are dearly missed.

Until we meet again.

Table of Contents

Table of Contents

Introduction

"What are little girls made of?" As the rhyme answers: "Sugar and spice and everything nice!" It seems that we girls with diabetes are made with *extra* sugar!

I have had type 1 diabetes for thirty-six years. When I was diagnosed in the mid-1970s, few people were familiar with what diabetes was. I didn't let that stop me. I always considered myself the "Johnny Appleseed" of diabetes education. Wherever I was and whenever I could, I would "plant seeds" of knowledge. First, I had to learn all the information that I could, which was available at that time. Then, I taught other people what diabetes was – like a spokesperson of this diabetes "club." It would be my fondest wish, if a cure were found, and put our club out of business. But, in the meantime, I continue on this journey to teach about diabetes. My path expanded beyond just teaching and became one of *helping* people with diabetes cope with the emotional issues of adjusting to diabetes.

Diabetes has become my life work! After many years of being an "unofficial" diabetes educator, I became an official Certified Diabetes Educator (CDE). As a clinical psychologist in private practice and a CDE, I feel that I am a good role model for my patients, as well as someone with a lot of empathy for the daily coping that people with diabetes must endure. I am able to successfully treat patients with diabetes with an understanding that comes from my own firsthand experience. My own personal philosophy is to take control of my diabetes and not let diabetes control my life. My focus strongly endorses empowering the lives of people with diabetes. My passion to teach about diabetes has been focused primarily on one-to-one (when not making presentations to diabetes groups). Now, via this book, I'm excited to continue to "plant" those seeds of knowledge about diabetes while reaching a larger audience!

This book assembles a very special collection of successful women with diabetes. Who better to share our ups and downs (with blood sugar or mood) than another woman who walks the same walk as us? Sometimes it helps just to know that other women have overcome the same challenges as we are going through. They can provide an inspiration to reassure us that we, too, can overcome the challenges we face.

Life for any woman can be challenging enough, but adding diabetes as an extra concern can leave someone feeling any assortment of emotional reactions: denial, anger, depression, guilt, or anxiety. But, when we see a woman with diabetes who manages to care for herself, as well as manage to care for her family and/or her career, we have to ask: "What's her secret to success?" In this book "*MY SWEET LIFE: Successful Women with Diabetes*" we get some answers to that question.

This book is not meant as a substitute for medical care. It is meant to enhance, encourage, empower, and educate you in your life journey with diabetes. It's important to understand that *we do the best we can* and it's okay not to be "perfect"! As you read through these life stories, you will find some common strategies for success among these women with diabetes. Successful women with diabetes have learned how to "make lemonade out of lemons" by accepting their illness and coping with it. They realize that, had it not been for their diabetes, they may not have chosen to live such a healthy lifestyle. Successful women with diabetes see this disease as "a blessing in disguise."

Just who are these women? They are a diverse group of highly-respected women – many of the contributing authors have type 1 diabetes, one has type 2, and a few have type 1.5/LADA (*Latent Autoimmune Diabetes in Adults*); with one exception, all of these women are insulin dependent. These women are diverse in geography – located on the East Coast, the West Coast, the Midwest, the South, and one is located "across the pond". These women range in ages from twenty-something to ninety years old. They also range in how many years they have had diabetes from a few years, to living well for seventy years! All these women have remarkably accomplished careers, some because of their diabetes, and some despite it.

Although each author's story is unique, there were many similarities among the women. One of the most common reactions to receiving a diagnosis of diabetes was the "Why me?" syndrome. That question was best answered by another question: Why not me? Many appreciated the fact that we are lucky to be diagnosed post-1921, when Drs. Banting and Best discovered insulin!

A recurrent theme that the contributing authors shared was their initial feeling of being alone with diabetes. Some had a sense of guilt or shame and tried to hide their illness. There was a prevailing feeling of not knowing anybody else to relate to, especially in those "dark ages" of diabetes care, before the advent of modern technology. Many of these women offered a "way out" to their boyfriends or husbands so they would not be trapped in a relationship with a partner who could end up with serious complications. The truly worthy man stayed with his woman and viewed the two working together as a team. These are blessed women to have found such wonderful men!

We are in a new age. Perceptions changed to recognize that we are not alone. Diabetes involves the whole family. Many of the women described how supportive their families were: mothers, especially, were seen as heroes. Family support also came from dads, brothers, sisters, grandparents, partners and children. Diabetes support can include friends, neighbors, and countrymen. So many women can now feel supported within the online diabetes community. Let's not forget the support we can receive from our diabetes medical team: doctors, nurses, nutritionists, diabetes educators, mental health professionals, and support groups, etc. There is no reason to ever feel alone anymore with your diagnosis. There are many sources of support available these days!

As you read these life stories, each woman shares her own pivotal moment when she came to an understanding of her own *empowerment*. Her inner strength is derived from a positive attitude about her ability to not just survive, but thrive, with diabetes. There's a moment in us all, arrived at in our own time, where we realize that life is what we make of it. We don't get the chance in life to choose the cards we are dealt. We do, however, get a choice in life to play the hand we have (or fold). These women are in the game and they are in it to win!

Their stories are heartwarming, as these women share their insights about finding balance between their body and mind, as well as in their personal, professional, and spiritual lives. This book is written for the newly-diagnosed woman who may need to learn some lessons of empowerment as she adjusts to her new lifestyle. Or, for the woman who has had diabetes for a while and would also benefit from uplifting, inspirational stories to encourage and motivate self-care. The title: "My Sweet Life" has the double connotation: one way it means *sweet* due to having *diabetes* and, the other way, *sweet* life means *enjoyable* life. The goal is for us to do both at the same time – live our lives with diabetes, but also enjoy our lives. It's a goal we can all strive toward!

So what can you learn from these women? If you have a positive attitude, you can appreciate the blessings in life. You can feel empowered to take control of your life. You can learn to have an attitude of gratitude, have a sense of humor and have respect for yourself. Live your life one day at a time, be mindful, and do your best. Maybe you can identify with just one story in this collection of twenty-four and relate it to yourself. That would be great! As they say: "live and learn." That would be my definition of a successful writer.

I'll leave you with this last quote, which Arthur Ashe, Jr. is credited with saying: "Success is a journey, not a destination." I wish all my diabetes sisters peace and love along their personal journey.

Beverly S. Adler, PhD, CDE

November 14, 2011
World Diabetes Day

Prologue

My Sweet Life

My sweet life means
I walk with pride
And keep my body strong.
My sweet life keeps me satisfied
By knowing right from wrong.
The blood that pulses
Through my veins
Is red and smooth and fine.
It carries all my nourishment
And it's uniquely mine.
For those of us
With sweeter blood
Our lives may go adrift.
But sweetness is a mighty flood,
And is, for us, a gift.
The gift is taking care of us.
We'll go to any length.
The gift may seem unfair to us,
But it's our source of strength.
So when you look at your sweet life
Be thankful you've been asked
To go through life as one who must
Perform this sweetest task.
To keep your organs clean and free
And ready for all strife.
And then, my friends,
You will be proud
To live
Your sweetest life.

Lorraine Brooks © 2011

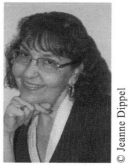

© Jeanne Dippel

Chapter 1   *by Beverly S. Adler, PhD, CDE*

Destiny's Plan: Diabetes is a Blessing in Disguise

The Beginning Phase

Who can say why I became a psychologist? Was it due to nature or nurture? This is a relevant question because I am the daughter of two very successful psychologists: Leonore Loeb Adler, PhD and Helmut E. Adler, PhD. Both of my parents have been influential in my life as a psychologist.

My mother always provided me with verbal encouragement, and was an assertive role model. She described herself as an early feminist, and espoused a philosophy of equal opportunities for men and women. She was highly motivated and goal oriented in her own endeavors and achievements. Because of her, I learned by observation that hard work and dedication make the difference between success and failure.

In my private practice, one goal for many of my female patients is to develop assertiveness in their lives, so they can optimize their opportunities. When women feel more in control of their lives, they subsequently feel less anxious and their self-esteem improves. This feeling of self-confidence and strength is one of the many lessons that I learned from my mother, and I am grateful to pass it on.

My father had a quieter influence in my life. He was a man of great knowledge, with an interest in many scientific and psychological topics. He was a gentle person and encouraged me in my education. Along the way, he and I enjoyed many lively academic discussions. Though he only rarely discussed it, I always knew that he was proud of my academic and professional achievements.

My inclination toward helping others in emotional distress started at a young age. When I was only five years old, I entered first grade. Under normal

1

circumstances, that event would have been memorable enough . But on this day, my mother walked me (and my little sister) to school in the midst of Hurricane Donna. When I got to school, I immediately started comforting the other kids. My mother reminded me of this many years later because she was so taken by this. Clearly, this was what I was destined to do, shown at its earliest phase.

The Day My Life Changed Forever

In 1974, I was in college, majoring in psychology. The fall semester of 1974 was rough, as I was taking an eighteen credit course load. It was very tiring, but I persevered and completed all the course requirements, earning A's and B's for my efforts. The next semester, Spring 1975, was again quite busy, as I took many tough courses. So at the time, it seemed natural that after such a hectic and stressful fall semester that I felt so totally exhausted.

My vision was blurry and my parents noticed a change in my energy level. I know they were deeply concerned, because I had all of the following problems: I had lost weight without dieting, I felt very thirsty all the time, and I was running to the bathroom to urinate frequently. I used to think to myself, *If I could drink the ocean, it still wouldn't be enough to quench my thirst!* That's why the route I took to all my classes followed every water fountain on campus. But despite all this, I was clueless that I was seriously ill.

In March of 1975, my parents, sister and I went to the family doctor's office because my sister needed a physician's signature for a school form. When my parents told the doctor that I had "lost the sparkle in my eyes," he immediately focused his attention on me. At the time, I thought my parents were crazy for saying that, and was very embarrassed that they had expressed their concerns to him. The doctor, though, agreed with my parents that something could be wrong and scheduled an appointment for me to return to his office for an oral glucose tolerance test. At this point, I was *still* clueless that anything was seriously wrong.

During my appointment (which had been made on the earliest possible date in the next week), I underwent the five-hour test. This involved drinking a sweetened drink and repeatedly taking my blood intravenousously. An appointment was scheduled to discuss the results on the following Friday. On that day, March 14, 1975, my life as I knew it changed forever. Because that was the day I was diagnosed with "juvenile diabetes."

How are you supposed to react to the news of being diagnosed with a chronic illness, one for which there is no cure?

In my family's case, there were all sorts of different reactions. My mother felt guilty, because she erroneously believed that had she and my father brought me to the doctor earlier, my diabetes could somehow have been prevented. (She was wrong; my parents were not responsible for my illness.) My sister was jealous, because at the time, she wore braces on her teeth. She told me that she wished she had the diabetes and I could have the braces. (Her logic was, "you can't see diabetes.") Of course, in due time, her braces were removed, her teeth were straight and her smile was beautiful, but I still had diabetes.

My brother had the most unique reaction of anyone that I have ever encountered in my entire life. His response after hearing the news about my diagnosis was to congratulate me! My brother explained this as follows: "Now I know that you will always take good care of yourself." My brother was right!

My own reaction to the diagnosis was rational, which allowed me to accept my illness very quickly. This was partly due to the fact that, at the same time as I underwent my five-hour glucose test, my mother had a student in one of her classes who was also ill, and, like me, went in for medical tests. When my mother's student's diagnosis came back as a brain tumor, it put my illness in perspective. Mine was a disease that I could live with!

Challenges

I had a different experience of adjusting to diabetes and learning about insulin shots than anybody else I know. Many people have told me that they found out about their diabetes only after being admitted into the hospital with high glucose readings. (I'm sure mine was also very high, but the doctor never told me my number!) Many people have also told me that they learned to inject insulin by first practicing on an orange. But not me!

During my follow-up appointment on Friday, my doctor (a General Practitioner), showed me how to take my first insulin injection by giving me my first shot. He explained that the needle needed to go into my thigh at a forty-five degree angle. Then, he told me to do the same thing to myself on Saturday.

The next day, I was terrified to give myself my own shot. So, I called the doctor, who told me to come into the office and he would demonstrate the procedure again. This time, however, he seemed annoyed. He told me that if I couldn't give myself the injection the next day (Sunday), I would have to call the Visiting Nurse Service because he would not be working. So, while I was still terrified to give myself an injection the next day, I did it.

My GP sent me to a diabetes specialist, Dr. Henry Dolger, for follow-up care. At the time, Dr. Dolger was very well-known for writing *the* book on diabetes, *HOW TO LIVE WITH DIABETES*. (I was fortunate enough to get an autographed copy of his book along with his gentle and supportive attention.) The first thing Dr. Dolger asked me to do was to demonstrate how I was injecting myself. When I reported that I was taking my shot at a forty-five degree angle into my thigh, as directed, he asked me, "Doesn't that hurt?"

I replied, "Why, yes, it does! Isn't it supposed to hurt?"

3

"No!" he answered. Then he taught me to inject at a ninety degree angle (perpendicular) into my thigh. Once I did this, I realized that he was right, because it felt so much less painful.

Over the course of time, the protocol for diabetes care, in general, has seen many changes due to all of the medical advances that have occurred. For example, when I was diagnosed in 1975, I used to take injections using disposable syringes (an improvement over the older glass syringes, which had to be boiled for sterilization). Today, I use an insulin pen for my insulin delivery. My first insulin regimen was one shot of long-acting insulin, per day. After a while, the regimen changed to two shots of long-acting insulin per day, which was the standard protocol.

Then came the Diabetes Control and Complications Trial (DCCT). The DCCT was a landmark medical study conducted from 1983 to 1993, and was funded by the National Institute of Diabetes and Digestive and Kidney Diseases that changed that standard protocol. This study showed that keeping blood glucose levels as close to normal as possible slows the onset and progression of the eye, kidney, and nerve damage caused by diabetes. The results of the DCCT demonstrated the success of four or more injections per day ("intensive insulin therapy") compared to the older approach of two or three shots per day.

My regimen was changed to this newer protocol of three shots of fast-acting insulin at each meal and a shot of long-acting insulin at bedtime. When people heard that I was now taking four shots of insulin per day, they expressed their sympathy because they believed that my diabetes had "worsened." I did my best to educate them that this regimen more closely approximated what a working pancreas did, and that the new regimen kept my blood sugar under better control. (Note that by my own choice, I have *not* moved on to the next advancement in insulin delivery, the insulin pump, which is a continuous infusion insulin delivery system.)

In 1975, the only way there was to tell how well you were controlling your blood sugar was by testing your urine. After you dipped a strip into the urine, it would change color to indicate how much sugar was being "spilled." This seems quite primitive compared to our current glucose meters, which measure blood glucose readings with far greater precision, but I didn't start using a glucose meter until the late 1980s when I was ready to start having children. In general, I currently check my blood glucose readings from eight to ten times per day in order to keep my blood sugar within target range.

New Challenges

Throughout my life, I have had to keep my attention focused on my diabetes. In general, my motto has always been to "take control of my diabetes and not let diabetes take control of me." After I earned two Master's degrees and a PhD degree, my career path was placed on hold as I focused my energy toward raising a family. My diabetes presented new challenges, though I refused to let diabetes restrict my life or my ability to have healthy children.

During my first pregnancy, I started using a glucose meter to check my blood sugar. I tended to be extremely vigilant during my pregnancies in order to maintain good control over my blood sugar. My obstetrician gave me a very nice compliment following the birth of my first child, when she said that my complication-free pregnancy was "as close to a non-diabetic pregnancy as possible". I had a second successful pregnancy in the early 1990s, and devoted myself to being a full-time Mommy.

Return to Career

After many years of childrearing, I was ready to return to my career. However, I was unsure what path to pursue.

My brother, in his wisdom, asked me, "If you had any wish, what would you like to do?"

I knew the answer to this without hesitation, so I told my brother that I would like to work with patients with diabetes. There was a Diabetes Education Center located near my home, and I was interested in working there. My brother's simple question has been the inspiration that guided me to the present. My brother's encouraging words to me, telling me to "go for it," have been my motivation to pursue that goal.

Through my family's pediatrician, I was given the name of the director of our local hospital's Mental Health Counseling Center. I called the director and scheduled an interview to discuss employment opportunities. Within weeks, I met with him. I explained with great enthusiasm my interest to work with patients who have diabetes.

He greeted my enthusiasm with the disappointing news that there was no behavioral medicine program at the Counseling Center with a specialty focus for patients with diabetes. I was not deterred by this news. I told him, "I would like to develop a program!" This pleased the director, so he hired me as a *per diem* staff psychologist.

While I worked on my own to develop a protocol for patients with diabetes, I became a specialist at treating patients with anxiety disorders. When my project was completed, I presented my new program to the director and the chief psychologist at the Counseling Center. My work primarily focused on involving the patients, who had many problems processing the emotional aspects of coping with diabetes (i.e., anger, denial, depression, stress and anxiety). I wanted to encourage and empower my patients with coping strategies in order to improve their adjustment. Three and a half years after that interview, I ran a successful therapy group at the hospital's Counseling Center, specifically tailored for patients with diabetes. As well, I maintained a caseload of patients in individual therapy for the treatment of anxiety and/or depressive disorders.

One of my favorite things to say to my patients who had low self-esteem was this: "Let me be your mirror." My intent was to help them see, through my perspective, what they had difficulty appreciating about themselves. One of my very special patients wrote a short poem about me and my approach to therapy:

"Let me be your mirror,
For I can plainly see,
All the great things about you,
Reflecting back at me."

This poem was very special to me because it reflected back to me how I was helping others. In this poem's simplicity, I found validation for the therapeutic work I invested in my patients.

In January of 2002, I took my career to the next level. In addition to my work at the Counseling Center, I started my own private practice. At first, it was only part-time. In 2004, due to the growth of my private practice, I left the Counseling Center in order to become a full-time private practitioner.

In 2002, I also became involved with the local (Baldwin) Lions Club, a chapter of the Lions Club International Foundation. Their focus on diabetes awareness and conquering blindness attracted me to their cause. Lions Clubs, in general, and the Baldwin Lions Club, in particular, are actively involved with providing services for the blind and visually impaired. Recycling eyeglasses is one of the Lions Club's most popular activities.

Our Baldwin Lions lend their support to the Lions Recycle for Sight Program. I do my part by keeping a collection box in my office, which ultimately gets added to other, donated used eyeglasses. Then, the eyeglasses are distributed to people who need them in developing countries, where they will have the greatest impact. I am also involved in fundraising activities such as our Strides: Lions Walk for Diabetes Awareness, which collects money to fund diabetes education for those who cannot afford to pay (note that diabetes education classes are often held in local hospitals). I served as our club's secretary from 2004 until 2010. Additionally, I served on the Lions Board of Directors for our Diabetes Education Center (in Nassau County, NY) from 2007 to 2009.

Presentations

In April of 2001, I was invited to participate at the 13th Annual Marriage and Family Therapy Conference as a panelist on a session devoted to the treatment of patients with diabetes and the role of family involvement. My paper was entitled, "Individual Psychotherapy Approach for the Treatment of the Diabetic Patient and the Role of Family Support." The emphasis of my presentation focused on the significant impact family members can have on the way a person with diabetes lives with his/her disease. With the addition of family support, a patient with diabetes can adapt to, and accept, the diagnosis of diabetes and his/her responsibility for self-care behaviors.

My reputation as a psychologist specializing in patients with diabetes began to grow as I made presentations at our local hospital's type 1 and/or type 2 support groups. One topic I presented was, "Changing Stinkin' Thinkin' to Smart Thinking: Learning How to Improve Coping with Diabetes using Cognitive Therapy Strategies," which focused on changing cognitive distortions into rational thinking. As well, I made presentations to a support group for parents of children/adolescents with diabetes at a local hospital's Diabetes Education Center. There, one topic I presented was, "Helping Your Diabetic Child or Teen Cope with Teasing and Bullies," which focused on children needing to be confident in order to stand up for themselves, their need to get involved with activities, and to be unafraid to join new groups, where the child or teen can gain a new set of friends who can also stand up for them.

In November of 2006, I was privileged to present the Keynote Address at the First Annual "Living with Diabetes - Dealing with the Day-to-Day Issues" one day educational seminar sponsored by the Juvenile Diabetes Research Foundation (JDRF) in Melville, NY. My topic was "'Psychoglycemia' – When Your Blood Sugar Goes Crazy." We know the correct word for high blood sugar is *hyperglycemia* and the correct word for low blood sugar is *hypoglycemia*. So, I created my own word, "psychoglycemia," to describe the craziness some people may feel in trying to manage the highs and lows of bouncing blood sugar.

In October of 2007, I was invited to make a presentation to the medical staff at a local hospital's Division of Endocrinology, Diabetes and Metabolism. My topic was, "The Psychology of the Noncompliant Patient with Diabetes." I identified psychological factors, such as stress, anxiety and depression, along with denial, which can affect compliance, as well as how providers can improve compliance by their actions as part of the "therapeutic partnership."

In March of 2008, I was again privileged to present the Keynote Address at the Second Annual Educational Seminar "Living with Diabetes," sponsored by the JDRF in Melville, NY. My presentation was entitled, "Type 1 Diabetes, Longevity and Mental Health." I spoke about how your attitude can make or break the balancing act of insulin, diet, and exercise needed to control diabetes. My message, then and now, is that having a positive attitude can help you live a longer, healthier, and happier life!

In March of 2010, I was a panelist at a "Tween" Scene Workshop for the JDRF Fourth Annual Educational Seminar in Melville, NY. My presentation topic was, "Safely Shifting Diabetes Care to your Tween," which focused on the role of the parents in encouraging the tween's gradual and progressive involvement in self-care with sensitivity, consistency, and empowerment.

Honors

I have received several honors for which I am very grateful as they acknowledge my achievements. Not all of the honors that I have received, though, have been related to my work with diabetes.

On September 11, 2001, I went to our local hospital and was prepared to help any patients suffering from trauma immediately following the attacks on the World Trade Center. I became involved with a program that came to be known as the Behavioral Health Trauma Response Team, where I worked on a weekly basis with individuals and families of the victims (heroes, all!) who died that day. The work was very emotional, as you might expect.

After one hundred-plus hours of service, I received a beautiful, framed copy of artwork (created by the art therapist who worked with the children who had attended the program) with a Certificate of Recognition for "Counseling friends and families in the aftermath of the World Trade Center tragedy." I felt proud, both of my service to these families to help them heal from their grieving, and to receive such an acknowledgement for my dedication to these families.

In 2007, I received the LillyforLife™ Achievement Award, sponsored by the Eli Lilly Pharmaceutical Company, in the category of "Professional Hero." I received a $1,500 cash prize and an etched trophy. I donated my cash award to my Baldwin Lions Club so they could continue their fine work in diabetes awareness.

In 2009, I was the recipient of the "Women of Distinction" award presented by Assemblyman Dave McDonough from the 19th Assembly District of New York for outstanding service to the community.

Most recently, I was extremely honored in 2010 to receive the "Melvin Jones Fellowship Award" presented from Lions Clubs International. It is their highest award, and was presented for my "Dedication to Humanitarian Service."

Certification as a Diabetes Educator

Since the earliest days, directly after my diagnosis, I have always felt like I was an unofficial diabetes educator because I set out to teach other people about diabetes. My professional focus was mainly on improving the emotional adjustment of patients, who were trying to cope with diabetes. So, it's not surprising that in 2009 I studied for the certification test to be an official Certified Diabetes Educator. After successfully passing this test, I was (and still remain) very proud to be a part of this "very small club," as William Polonsky, PhD, CDE and Chief Executive Officer at the Behavioral Diabetes Institute called it, of practicing "diabetes psychologists" in the United States.

Publications

In 2004, I sent a letter to *Diabetes Forecast* magazine in response to an article they published. Two months later, I was very happy to see *my* letter in print while reading the newest edition's "Mail Call" section.

Several years passed before I tried writing again. I was inspired to write following an assembly for students at our local middle school, which I attended, with a guest speaker who published children's books. His presentation was geared toward the kids, as he told them to follow their dream of writing and not to give up. His message was a hit with me, so I decided to try to write something new.

This time, I wrote an article that was inspired due to an idea I had during a session with one of my patients. He was a newly-diagnosed eighteen-year-old man. He was overwhelmed, angry, and uncooperative with regards to his diabetes management.

Since this young man had also recently gotten his driver's license, I tried to break down the different aspects of taking care of yourself by making comparisons to driving a car. I made analogies such as, "Checking your speedometer to maintain your speed within the legal limit is like checking your blood glucose to keep it within the target range." And, "Your blood glucose reading is like checking your gas gauge; it provides information such as whether your gas tank is low and you need to fill up." The analogy went on to compare eating well with using the correct gasoline in the car's gas tank and that reading food labels is like paying attention to road signs. I also made the comparison that changing the oil every three months to keep the car "healthy" was like having your A1C checked every three months for a person with diabetes to stay healthy.

My message (and title of my article) was, "You're in the Driver's Seat: Caring for your Diabetes." I submitted my article for publication, and it was accepted in the American Association of Diabetes Educators' publication *in Practice* as a "practice pearl." The success of this article validated that my ideas have merit. Writing has provided me with another avenue in which to share my message of empowerment.

Diabetes as a Blessing in Disguise

What I could have seen as a terrible diagnosis of type 1 diabetes, thirty-six years ago, has actually been a blessing in disguise![1] I wonder where I would be today, if my life had not changed so much on March 14, 1975?

I think my brother had the right idea; when I was first diagnosed, he congratulated me, certain that I would take good care of myself from then on. He was right, as I *do* take good care of myself. More than that, I have not only lived with my own diabetes for many years, but I have helped (and continue to help) so many *other* people who also live with diabetes.

In my private practice, I focus on strongly endorsing and empowering the lives of people with diabetes. I believe that I am a good role model for my patients, as well as someone who has a lot of empathy with regards to the daily routine of coping that people with diabetes must face. Because of my own, firsthand experience, I have been able to successfully treat others who struggle with diabetes. I love what I do and feel that I am uniquely qualified to treat patients with diabetes.

Many of the people I see have to deal with many emotional challenges before they are able to accept that they've been diagnosed with diabetes. I think the most difficult age group to work with is comprised of teenagers. Teenagers quite naturally seek autonomy during this stage of life and don't want to accept parental guidance. But I have the key to open a dialogue with them, because I not only "talk the talk, but I walk the walk." Or, in other words, I know about the ups and downs of living with diabetes (quite literally). Because of that, teens are more willing to accept my help.

Now, let's return to the original question I posed at the beginning of this chapter: "Who can say why I became a psychologist?" I think the answer is part nature and part nurture, but mostly destiny. I believe that I was born with the gifts, talents, and abilities that I would need in life. I feel my purpose here, in the grand scheme of the Universe, is to help others.

I believe that *everyone* is born with a purpose, although we may not necessarily recognize just what that purpose is. I think I have become the person I was meant to be due to acquiring the special set of skills I would need in this life, then applying them in order to help others. In so doing, I've taken what is seen by some as the "lemons" in life, and turned it into lemonade.

When people who don't know me well express their sympathy that I have diabetes, I tell them with a smile that they should not be sad for me. Diabetes is an illness that I can *live* with, and control (to a certain extent). I haven't missed

---

1 I realize that not everyone may feel the same way I do. I fully respect the rights of others to feel differently.

out on *anything* in life due to my diabetes. On the contrary – you could say that diabetes has been *good* to me. I take care of myself, and it's the basis for my career. In that way, I'm happy to have diabetes.

As life unfolds, one may understand "destiny's plan" more clearly. You can embrace it or you can curse it, but you *can't* change it. You need to say to yourself, "These are the cards I've been dealt," and deal with it.

In my case, I can't answer *why* it is so that I have diabetes. I have chosen to accept that this is part of what my life is, in order to move forward along the road to being the best me that I can be. You might even say that having diabetes is one of the reasons why I'm so sweet! (Just kidding.)

Website: www.AskDrBev.com

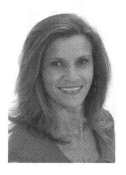

Chapter 2   *by Brandy Barnes, MSW*

It's All About
Perspective . . .

The nurse walked into the exam room and announced that all of my lab work came back clear. She told me I was free to go, and that the doctor would be in soon with my paperwork to check out. A sense of relief washed over me. Glancing over at my mom, I saw the stress leave her face and I knew that she, too, was happy with the nurse's words.

Suddenly, the door swung open. We were jolted back into reality by the doctor, who said, "I'm sorry. There's been a terrible mistake. You *do* have diabetes and you need to go directly to the hospital. We've already called ahead and they are expecting you." He told me that my blood sugar was 450 mg/dL, dangerously high, and I could be close to *diabetic ketoacidosis*; hence the urgency in getting me to the hospital.

Before leaving the room, he offered me a diet Coke. Although I was dying of thirst, the thought of drinking a diet Coke was repulsive, so I shook my head with an emphatic "no."

"Are you sure you don't want one?" he asked. "This is what you will have to get used to drinking. No more sugary soft drinks."

Eventually, a nurse came in and placed a cup of icy diet Coke on the counter in the exam room. If looks could have killed that drink, it would have been dead!

In a state of disbelief, I thought, What? How can this be happening?

At the exact same moment, the emotional roller coaster ride that my mom had been on since the nurse had walked in hit an even higher peak as I saw tears well up in her eyes. Silence reigned as we retreated into our own heads to figure out how to handle the life-changing news that had just been dropped into our laps.

At the time, I was a sophomore in high school and only fifteen years old. I had so much ahead of me, and I had big plans. I was either going to be a famous broadcast journalist like Barbara Walters or I was going to have my own talk show like Oprah. How would diabetes fit into those big plans?

Although I was surprised, I have to admit that the news wasn't a complete shock. Just the night before, my mom had noticed how much water I was drinking (in light of the fact that I did not particularly like water) and commented on it. When she went into her bedroom, she started whispering with my dad.

I followed her in and promptly asked, "What are you talking about? What do you think is wrong with me?"

She replied, "It's probably nothing, but we'll just go to the doctor and have them check you out tomorrow."

"No!" I shouted. "I want you to tell me what you think it is!"

"Well, you know your dad's sister, JoAnn, has diabetes," my Mom replied. "We just want to make sure you don't have it."

My mind started to race. I left the room and started to research this disease, *diabetes*, that I knew virtually nothing about. After finding the symptoms in one of my parents' books, my heart sank. I had almost every one of them.

The date was January 21, 1990. It is a date that will be forever ingrained in my mind. That's the date that life as I knew it changed forever, because it's the date I was diagnosed with diabetes.

After I was admitted to the hospital, I was hooked up to IVs, flat on my back in the hospital bed and staring straight ahead at the wall. The nurses came in to talk with me, but I remained non-responsive and just kept staring straight ahead. I remember hearing my mom outside the door saying to a nurse, "I'm getting worried about her."

To provide a little more perspective about what was going on in my life prior to my diagnosis: six months before, I had returned from a life-altering three-week journey to the Ukraine with twenty-four other high school students. The Ukraine had just begun its struggle for independence from the Soviet Union, so I had seen first-hand how difficult life *could* be. We spent the time overseas with Ukrainian families, including some who were members of the Communist Party. Most of the people we interacted with had never seen or spoken with an American before.

Once I returned to school, I was on the newspaper staff and played three sports. My family was an average American household of two working parents and two daughters. There was a seven year gap between me and my younger sister, Candace.

My journey with diabetes began just before Christmas in December of 1989, when I came down with the flu over Christmas break. In the weeks after my recovery, I continued to lose weight. Since I had always been very thin and not a big eater, my mom was concerned about my continued weight loss. To combat the weight loss, in January, my mom started preparing chocolate milkshakes for me every morning before school. (Little did she know the devastating impact this was having on my blood sugar level - hindsight is always 20/20!)

Since my diagnosis was in January, it was the middle of the high school basketball season and I was a key player on our junior varsity basketball team. Just a few days prior to my diagnosis, I had asked a friend to sit behind the bench at our game with the biggest cup of Coke that could be found, and to refill it when the liquid level got low. Also, during biology class in the week prior to my diagnosis, I had noticed that my vision was blurry when I looked across the hall. I mentioned my concern to my friends, but then I just shook it off as nothing important. All of these telltale signs came back to me when the nurse started explaining the signs and symptoms of high blood sugar.

Although we all go through the five stages of grief at different rates, I think I went through at least four (denial, anger, bargaining, and depression) while lying in the hospital bed that first day. This was part of the natural progression through the stages, including the often asked question, "Why me?"

I was relieved when the "Man Above" graciously sent one of my mom's friends, Cindy, into my room with an answer that same day. I'll never forget her words. She said, "Brandy, God would never give you more than you could handle."

At first, I sarcastically thought, *Ahhh! So, I got this disease because I am strong. What a great reward!* But further contemplation led me to a feeling of pride and empowerment. I later thought, *Hmmm . . . I guess that means that I'm pretty strong . . . .pretty fierce then, huh?* It also made me think about the purpose of my diagnosis, but I'll talk more about that later.

Then I thought about a friend from school who had recently been through a health challenge; she had seemed to disappear afterward. She was still in school, but she had shrunk away into a shell of herself. I knew that I could not let diabetes do this to me.

First, I needed to get answers to my burning questions: Would I be able to continue playing basketball this season, or ever again, for that matter? Would I still be able to play softball or run cross country? How would I tell my friends at school, and how would they react?

No one else in my school had diabetes, so there was no map for me to follow. So while I knew this diagnosis was going to change my life, I just wasn't sure what that change entailed.

15

The first couple of days in the hospital were all about self-examination. It was while I was lying in bed, deeply entrenched in soul-searching, that I came to a pivotal realization. This thought would be so important that it would significantly impact how I dealt with challenges for the rest of my life, yet it was also very simple. My thought was, *It's all about perspective.*

There is a famous quote from Charles R. Swindoll that says, "Life is 10% what happens to you and 90% how you react to it." Until this diagnosis, which was the biggest challenge I had ever faced in my life, those words had held little meaning. But now, I suddenly got it! I had no say (none) in whether or not I would have this disease, nor did I know why it had been forced on me. That was the 10%. But like many people, when life started to spin out of control, I started grasping for whatever I could in a vain search for stability.

I felt so much relief when I realized that here, what I could control was *me*, along with my reaction to this diagnosis. Within myself, I had the ability to shape my experience with this disease as a blessing, or a curse. That was the ever-important 90% that Swindoll had referenced. It was a simple, yet powerful, concept.

Although I was young, I understood that I stood at a crossroads in my life. I had a decision to make about how I was going to view this disease, much less how I wanted others to view me with this disease.

On the second day of my hospital stay, I was greeted by one of my basketball teammates, Karla. She came not as a visitor, but as my roommate! At first, I'd honestly thought the nurse was joking when she asked if I minded having Karla as a roommate, but she wasn't. Karla had been admitted to the hospital due to asthma.

We spent a lot of time over the next few days bonding over our chronic illnesses. What made the experience more fun was the fact that all of our friends from school came to visit us. In a sense, we had "the cool hospital room" because we always had lots of visitors.

The rest of high school was pretty uneventful. I continued to play softball, basketball, and to run cross country, and went on to be the editor of my high school newspaper. I even traveled abroad with a school group during the summer of my junior year.

As the only person in my high school with diabetes, I felt deeply obligated to represent diabetes in a positive way because my experience was the only picture many of my classmates were likely to have of the disease, aside from an occasional grandparent or aunt. But uncovering the purpose for my disease remained a constant thought, one that nagged me in the back of my mind.

In college, I spread my wings, hoping to find that elusive friend with diabetes who would understand what life was like for me. This need to be understood by a friend with diabetes was something I had never experienced, but it was something I definitely longed for, more than I realized at the time. Unfortunately, this friend was nowhere to be found on the big campus of the University of North Carolina (UNC) at Chapel Hill; at least, she wasn't in any of the places I looked.

I volunteered to lead UNC's Student Diabetes Support Group and took an internship promoting healthy living on campus, hoping to find her in one of those places. Unfortunately, it didn't take long to realize that college was not the time or place when most people wanted to disclose their diabetes to their peers. They were even less likely to want to go to a support group and talk about it for an hour.

When a new endocrinologist came to town to start the new diabetes program at UNC, I wasted no time in registering as a patient. My diabetes journey would have two new, important experiences that would play out in this new endocrinologist's office. The first event occurred when I discovered that the Certified Diabetes Educator, Camille, had diabetes. The connection between us was immediate! Ahhh! It felt so good to finally find another woman with diabetes. Now I had someone to share funny diabetes stories with, and someone to ask those questions that could only be answered by a woman who had been there and done that – with diabetes! That experience was monumental, as it caused me to wonder if there were any other women with diabetes out there who longed for this same kind of connection.

The other life-altering experience that happened was that I had a lot of in-depth conversations with the endocrinologist, John Buse, MD, PhD, regarding my career path. Although it is not the norm to spend your visit to the endocrinologist discussing your career path, it was exactly what I needed at the time. Dr. Buse's unwavering view was that people with diabetes were no different than anyone else; in hearing him state that over and over again, I started to believe it, too. At the time, I had no idea what a big role he would play in my career development over the next twenty years, as his encouragement helped push me into pursuing a career in diabetes.

During the spring of my junior year of college, I reluctantly went on an insulin pump. I was very self-conscious about wearing the pump outside of my clothing. I felt like I was walking around with a sign that said, "I am wearing an insulin pump. Ask me what it does!" While I had never been ashamed of my diabetes, I also didn't want to walk around with a big sign on saying, "I have diabetes." I liked having the ability to reveal my diabetes whenever I wanted to and the pump took some of that control away from me. I must admit that I even had a few bouts of inconsolable crying due to not being able to wear a favorite dress with the pump. But, after I got used to it, I conceded that life was much better on the pump, and so was my blood sugar!

It was shortly after I went on the pump that I met Chris, the man I would later marry. Our initial conversations didn't involve diabetes because, as he later disclosed, he thought my insulin pump was a pager. Chris stood out because he was kind, gentle, open-minded and didn't pry too much about my diabetes. (In other words, my assessment of the possibility of him turning into the "diabetes police" came back negative!) He was truly interested in learning about me as a person, and he viewed diabetes as a part of me that made me, well, myself. He also stood out because he showed concern about my diabetes, but never worry or fear.

Throughout my senior year of college, Chris and I spent more and more time together. He began to recognize when my blood sugar was low and even helped me through a few really bad lows. He saw first-hand what life was like for a woman with diabetes and I saw first-hand that he was "a keeper."

Shortly after graduating from college, I disclosed my post-college work plans to Dr. Buse during one of my check-up visits. My plan was to work (to support myself) while also attending graduate school in a diabetes-related field. By this time, I had come to think of Dr. Buse as a mentor. I was pleasantly surprised when he offered to hire me to work at his clinic, if I got into graduate school, to pursue a career in the diabetes field. It could have very well been a flippant comment on his part, but I took him very seriously.

Ironically, I received my acceptance letter into the UNC School of Social Work the day before a scheduled follow-up visit with him. I shared my plans to address the emotional needs of people with diabetes by becoming a social worker. When I showed him my acceptance letter, he kept his word.

By the fall, I was working full-time as a Clinical Trials Coordinator on the American Diabetes Association's GENNID trial at his clinic. This study was aimed at gaining a better understanding of the genetics involved in the development of type 2 diabetes.

Over the next three years, I worked full-time and went to school part-time to earn my Master's degree in Social Work (with a concentration in health care settings). Our shared goal was for me to be the Social Worker at the UNC Diabetes Care Center and Dr. Buse frequently reminded me that I was "blazing new trails in the field of diabetes" because there were no known social workers with diabetes who worked in any diabetes clinics.

I guess I should have seen that as a bit of a red flag. But I had seen Dr. Buse seemingly create jobs out of thin air, so the thought that it would not happen again didn't occur to me as I was young and naïve. My dream came to a screeching halt about one month prior to graduation, when Dr. Buse came to me and said, "I have some bad news. The hospital can't figure out how to be reimbursed for social work services in a clinic setting, so the only way you can work here is if you work for free."

For many people, this kind of news could have been devastating after working toward a specific goal for three years. But my diabetes diagnosis had prepared me for situations like this. From my diagnosis, I learned that life doesn't always go as planned – even when you have the best plans in place. I also learned that, "*it's all about perspective!*"

So my career path took a slight detour, as I went to work at the American Cancer Society as a marketing/program manager. It was around this time that Chris proposed to me after five years of dating. Of course, no diabetes proposal would be complete without a good *hypoglycemia* story to go with it!

The night of October 5, 2001, started out like a typical Friday evening. This was just after the horrible events of September 11, 2001, and we were still coming to terms with the short- and long-term effects of our national tragedy. It had certainly made me take a deep look at what was important in life, and I think it had a similar effect on Chris. Chris spent the entire week prior to October 5 practicing my favorite romantic song at the time, "*For You*" by Kenny Lattimore. (Chris is a natural singer!)

On the night of my proposal, I went upstairs to take a shower and left him downstairs watching television. As I was getting out of the shower, I could tell that my blood sugar was low. So, I quickly dried off, dressed, and headed downstairs to treat my low. When I got about halfway down the stairs, I realized that all of the lights were off. Suddenly, Chris started singing. I immediately turned toward him and saw the candles and flowers and realized that he was singing to me! I could tell he had spent a lot of time making sure everything looked and sounded perfect, so, being the nice Southern girl that I am, I decided not to interrupt him to tell him that my blood sugar was low!

It took a minute for it to register why he was doing all of this. But even after I started to put it together, I didn't equate how long the song was. Nor did I think about the time involved in him getting down on one knee to tell me how much I had come to mean to him over the last five years. Needless to say, by the time he got to: "Will you marry me?" I was a blubbery mess! I was sweating and I couldn't think of what I was supposed to say to him. (You know what it's like when your blood sugar gets so low that someone could ask you a simple question like, "What is 1 +1?" and you just cannot, for the life of you, think of the right answer!)

As Chris tells the story, there was a very long, agonizing silence before I finally said, "My blood sugar is low. I need something!" Eventually, he got his answer after I drank some juice! (The answer was "yes," of course. But then, that's just a typical day in the life of a woman with diabetes, right?)

In 2003, I decided to leave the nonprofit world and venture into the corporate world to sell diabetes products for a pharmaceutical company. Although I had learned a great deal and enjoyed my experiences at the American

Cancer Society, I knew my passion was to help others with diabetes, especially because I still hadn't uncovered my purpose for having this disease. In August of 2003, I took a job as a sales representative in Raleigh, North Carolina with Aventis Pharmaceuticals. It took a lot of hard work to get the job and I remember feeling very proud when the job was offered, as I was ready to prove myself in corporate America.

I was a natural when it came to talking about diabetes. The medical staff was equally enamored by the fact that I had diabetes and was selling diabetes medications. They asked me all kinds of questions, and I felt especially empowered when doctors would say, "You're more of an expert on diabetes than I am because you live with it all day, every day. I could probably learn a few things from you!"

Wow! I thought, *maybe this was the purpose behind my diabetes.* Although I wasn't interacting with patients as I had originally dreamed, I was teaching the doctors (who treat them) about diabetes and sharing some important lessons with them along the way.

During my six years as a pharmaceutical sales representative, I learned a lot about running my own business. I even won a few sales awards. The aspect of the job that I did not enjoy was the "pressured sell" or the "hard sell." I preferred to sell with a consultative approach that included a lot of dialogue, rather than a monologue that involved me spitting out facts about the products I was selling.

Because of my interest in psychology, I wanted to get to know the physicians and build a strong relationship, so they could trust the information I was sharing with them. I also wanted to make it clear that my priority was the patient with diabetes (because I was a patient with diabetes myself). Then, rather than feeling like they were being "sold to," it would be a consultative visit. They learned which patients would benefit most from using my products and the best approaches for motivating patients. The best part was that I had purposely selected a company whose products I had used and believed in. (The job would have been impossible for me otherwise!)

In love and on top of the world, Chris and I decided to embark on the pregnancy journey about two years after getting married. Based on the numerous infertility stories in the news, I was somewhat worried about how long it would take me to become pregnant. We were pleasantly surprised to find out that I was pregnant in August of 2004 with a due date of April 15, 2005.

I experienced all of the normal highs of being pregnant for the first time, but I also felt some lows that aren't experienced by women who aren't living with diabetes. Having a healthy baby, for an expectant mom who has pre-existing diabetes, takes a lot of work – lots more blood sugar testing, lots more doctor visits, lots more weigh-ins and blood pressure monitoring, and lots more people in my business – poking and prodding me all the time. This was when I really needed that female friend with diabetes. I looked on the Internet, looked for resources in my local community, and even asked my high-risk obstetrician and my endocrinologist, but I was unable to connect with another woman who had been through a successful pregnancy with diabetes. So, I spent a lot of time worrying if what I was experiencing was normal.

After my beautiful, healthy daughter named Summer was born on April 12, 2005, I thought about the significant efforts I had put into finding resources during my pregnancy. I was disappointed and angry that there were so few resources available for women with diabetes at times when we needed them the most. I knew there had to be other women out there with diabetes who felt the same way.

Although 2007 started off fine, it went downhill quickly. In March, I was hospitalized due to a kidney stone. Exactly a month later, I was back in the hospital with severe stomach pain resulting from appendicitis. Then, one month later, I was again hospitalized after I started vomiting one night and couldn't stop. Even at the hospital, heavy medications couldn't stop the dry heaving. Finally, after three days in the hospital, I was discharged with no diagnosis.

After several hospital stays and rapid weight loss, my mom pushed me to get to the bottom of what was going on with me. So I called my trusted endocrinologist, Dr. Buse, and asked him to test me for "everything." Although he thought I was being a bit dramatic, he followed my wishes and when my results came back, everything was normal except my calcium level. I went back in to have it re-tested and then found out that I had *hyperparathyroidism*.

"What is that?" you ask. (Indeed; I asked the same thing!)

I found out that we have four parathyroids that surround our thyroid, and one of mine was "bad" or malfunctioning. Since parathyroids regulate your calcium level, it was this lack of regulation that had caused calcium to leak over into my urine and create the kidney stone I had endured a few months prior. It was likely the parathyroid had also caused the vomiting episode. The appendicitis was just a bonus. (Ha!).

Of course, I had to undergo surgery to remove the "bad" parathyroid. So, in September of 2007, the surgery took place. I can honestly say that I felt like I had a new lease on life as soon as I woke up from the surgery. Physically, I felt like a new person, too!

Not only was my body healed, but my mind was clearer. I began to feel a very strong internal pull on my soul. It is hard to describe, but I felt like I was being called to do more to help people with diabetes using all of the blessings and gifts I had received in life. Although I once thought that pharmaceutical sales could be my calling, I now understood that it was one of the stages of progress toward uncovering my purpose. So, I tried various things to figure out what my purpose was – from praying, to reading motivational books, to taking "strength finder" tests.

As fate would have it, a vision came to me one sunny day in the Fall of 2007 while driving down I-95 to my first appointment of the day. I immediately pulled off the interstate and wrote everything down on a legal tablet in my car. Then, I sat back and looked at the tablet.

"Weekly blogs," "buddy program," "columns from experts who are living with diabetes," "a forum for women to talk to each other," "a store where women with diabetes can purchase items made specifically for them," and "an annual retreat" were some of the things written on the tablet. Immediately, I thought it was a great idea. I knew I would have loved to have had access to this kind of resource over the last seventeen years, especially when I was pregnant.

I also thought about how much work it would be. As a wife, mother of a two-year-old, and full-time employee, I couldn't see a way that there would be time for a project so big. So, I went home and put the tablet in the back of my desk and hoped it would just go away. But, as the days and weeks went by, I found myself thinking about and planning ways to make it happen. I was giddy with excitement when I thought about the huge impact it could have on women with diabetes in my community, my state, the nation, and even the world.

In November, I took the tablet to my husband and began explaining what I felt God had revealed to me as my purpose. As only a truly supportive husband could, he stopped me before I could finish and excitedly said, "What are you doing sitting here?!? This is what you should be doing! You need to be doing this!"

DiabetesSisters.org, a national nonprofit organization whose mission is to improve the health and quality of life of women with and at risk of developing diabetes, and to advocate on their behalf, became a reality – the Website was launched on January 31, 2008. Over the next two years, my life became more and more consumed with DiabetesSisters as more people learned about us. The organization expanded to include lots more for women with diabetes, including nationwide support groups called PODS (Part of DiabetesSisters) Meetups, and a very innovative SisterMatch Program.

After a successful collaboration with Dr. Steve Edelman and Sandy Bourdette of Taking Control of Your Diabetes (TCOYD) in Raleigh, NC in 2009, DiabetesSisters began working toward making the "annual retreat" a reality. To my complete amazement, the first annual Weekend for Women Conference hosted by DiabetesSisters and TCOYD took place on May 22-23, 2010 – a little over two years after the idea was written down on that legal note tablet! Women with all types of diabetes ranging in ages from twenty to eighty-one years old flew in from twenty-one states to attend!

What very few people knew was how challenging the year prior to the conference had been for me on a personal level. At the same time that I had started doing major fundraising for the first ever Weekend for Women Conference, I had to schedule surgery to remove my enlarged thyroid (goiter) as it had been causing difficulty swallowing. The surgery went well, except that my thyroid levels were in need of adjustment. This imbalance made me incredibly lethargic and unable to concentrate, but I learned that the thyroid medication had to be titrated very slowly.

When I went in for my follow-up visit with the surgeon in October, I heard the words that no one wants to hear: "You have cancer." Although it was surreal, I chose to focus on the fact that it was one of the slowest-growing and least deadly forms of cancer. I considered myself blessed. My radioactive iodine treatment was scheduled for after the holidays since it required a low iodine diet for two weeks prior.

I was working on making the conference a reality when I was faced with another huge challenge the following month. In October, I received a frantic phone call from my mom. "The doctors think your dad has cancer again," she said with a shaky voice. My dad had already beaten cancer (Hodgkin's disease) once during my senior year of high school. This time, his diagnosis was more complicated and took a number of failed biopsies and a surgery at Duke University Medical Center to finally determine the type of cancer it was. I was heavily involved in getting my father diagnosed correctly and determining the best form of treatment for him.

Throughout the entire ordeal, I kept praying, "Please don't let it be pancreatic cancer; anything but that. Please." When the results came back, that it was a rare combination of two forms of cancer, but highly "treatable," I jumped for joy. In my mind, as long as my father didn't have pancreatic cancer, we could handle anything.

The reality was that I was blessed, and it would be foolish to see it any other way. I could drown in the sorrow of me and my dad having cancer, or I could be thankful for everything I had, including my own life and my dad. My dad underwent intensive chemotherapy for six months and was in his fourth treatment when the Weekend for Women Conference took place the following May.

While I may have been ready to move on from the difficult year of 2009, 2009 wasn't quite finished with me. I finished out the year by being laid off from my full-time job in pharmaceutical sales just before Christmas. This was the point where I began to feel a bit demoralized. Thankfully, with the support of my husband, Chris, I was able to remain calm and give some deep consideration to my career plans. He repeatedly told me not to think about the loss of income, but instead to really think and pray about what I wanted my future to look like.

The answer to my prayers came pretty quickly. By January of 2010, sponsorship checks for the 2010 Weekend for Women Conference started rolling in. By the end of the month, I had collected enough money to cover the entire conference and a small salary for me in 2010.

2010 started with a fresh new perspective and a brand new full-time job. Although I was used to being out in doctors' offices and conversing with people face-to-face every day, I quickly adapted to working from home. I also discovered that devoting 100% of my work time to DiabetesSisters opened many more opportunities. I now had time to explore new funding and partner relationships, as well as consider new projects that I would never have been able to even think about when DiabetesSisters was not my full-time job.

Wow! It really felt like my life had come full circle. All of my education (Bachelor's degree in Psychology and Master's Degree in Social Work) and all of my previous jobs – from clinical research in diabetes to nonprofit program management at the American Cancer Society to sales and marketing in the diabetes pharmaceutical world – had all happened for a very important reason . . . to provide the skills necessary to lead a national nonprofit organization for women with diabetes.

This was what I had been working toward all along! This was my purpose, and my true calling!

This was confirmed at the conclusion of the 2010 Weekend for Women Conference, when I sat in a room full of women with diabetes, heard many random beeps from meters and pumps, and observed the smiling faces of women as they connected with other women like they had never done before. This was exactly what I had envisioned back in 2007!

Although you often hear that conference/event planning is a thankless job, I am honored to say that women with diabetes are some of the most grateful people on earth. I have never in my life heard the words "thank you" as many times as I did that weekend! The surveys that the women completed also told the real story. "I have looked for something like this for so long. I am so glad to finally have the support that I have needed for the last thirty years" and "This conference saved my life. I was at the end of my rope . . . out of ideas and out of hope. This conference showed me that I am not alone in this disease. I have a whole Sisterhood. And I have new strategies to use to manage my diabetes better," were just a few of the comments.

The success of the conference spread quickly through the diabetes community. The following month (June), I found myself in a meeting with Dr. Bill Polonsky discussing the idea of partnering with The Behavioral Diabetes Institute to bring the Conference to the West Coast. The rest of the summer was a whirlwind of conferences, meetings, and speaking engagements.

It has been full throttle since the first conference in May of 2010, with little time to rest. My entire family has gotten involved in the organization in various ways to show their support, which has been a godsend. At the first conference, my sister, Candace, immediately stepped in to handle the Registration Desk and help with Onsite Operations. My husband, Chris, stepped in as the Onsite Operations Manager and received standing ovations from the attendees at the Conference. He was the only male involved in the Conference, so it could have been awkward. Instead, women came up to both of us and told us how inspirational it was to see us working together on a cause that meant so much to both of us.

To take it one step further, after observing spouses standing around in the hallways waiting for their wives and talking to them, Chris decided that he wanted to give back even more by leading a program for the spouses at the next Conference. As he pointed out, spouses and significant others rarely have anyone to talk to about the ups and downs of living with a woman with diabetes. Not to be left out, my daughter, Summer, who is now six years old, informed me that she would like to perform Alicia Keys' song *Superwoman* as a gift to the women at the next conference. She would also like to hold a session on "what it's like to be the child of a woman with diabetes." Pretty insightful for a six-year-old!

At thirty-six years of age, I am in a good place. I went through a lot to get to this point. There were lots of ups and downs, but I kept a positive outlook because I learned early on that *it is all about perspective*. Some people say that if they could have one wish it would be to take away their diabetes. I, on the other hand, do not feel that way at all.

Diabetes has made me who I am today. It has taken me on many journeys and I have experienced many things that I would not have experienced otherwise. Without diabetes, I would have never met so many amazing innovators in the diabetes field, nor would I have met so many phenomenal women with diabetes! Diabetes has also made me stretch myself into uncomfortable areas – including public speaking and Web development – things that I would not have done if I was not so passionate about diabetes.

Rather than focusing on the numerous illnesses, surgeries, and challenges, I choose to be thankful for all I have and focus on the many blessings I have received. Thinking about it any other way would make life less enjoyable – and I want all the joy I can possibly have in this life!

Website: www.diabetessisters.org

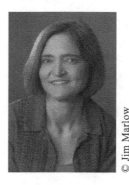
© Jim Marlow

Chapter 3   *by Claire Blum, MS Ed, RN, CDE*

Living on the Edge

My life has always been an adventure. Even when I was very young, I enjoyed living life on the edge . . . literally!

Thirty minutes before my oldest sister's graduation from high school, while my Mother and Grandmother picked flowers along the side of the road, I was off exploring a trail that meandered around a nearby cave. When I saw them preparing to move on, I began to run in an attempt to catch up. This might be why I didn't notice when the trail took a sharp turn. Looking ahead, it appeared as though jumping over a gentle slope would allow me to land on the trail again. With less than a second to react, I bent my knees and jumped . . . 14 feet to the road below. I have always believed that my guardian angel helped me see a much gentler slope of the cliff than was actually there, as I'd have surely fallen to my death if I hadn't jumped over the edge. Both heels were broken, but my life was spared.

My life with type 1 diabetes began in much the same style . . . by jumping in, figuring out what needed to be done, and doing it.

In 1978 at the age of 17, my parents moved to the Far East. I spent the fall semester in Korea, adapting to cultural change and life in a Third World country. Over the Christmas holiday, I became deathly ill with pneumonia, persistent cough, and severe headaches. By early January, I was sent off to join other missionary kids at a school in Singapore. But I continued to cough, and struggled to bounce back to my usual energetic self. My weight dropped, and I was constantly thirsty, making frequent trips to the bathroom. My legs began to cramp, and my dear, sweet roommate would often get up during the night to rub them in hopes of relieving the pain.

Around that time and unbeknownst to me, my older sister, still living in the United States, had been diagnosed with type 1 diabetes. My mother sent word to the school nurse, asking her to have me tested.

On April 6, 1978, a day I remember clearly, I got up early to go to the local hospital. They had me drink a "sugary cocktail," then began to draw my blood every thirty minutes. It was quickly apparent that the technicians had minimal training, as they jabbed and dug, sometimes for several minutes, to draw blood from my arms.

When the testing was finally over, I was released back to school. As I stood in the hall, waiting for class to begin, it seemed that my energy level was at an all time low. I thought to myself, *How can a person feel so badly after sitting around and doing nothing?* Minutes later, the school nurse appeared and told me that I needed to return to the hospital.

After arriving at the hospital for the second time that day, a doctor advised me that I had diabetes. My blood glucose had gone over 400 mg/dL during the glucose tolerance test, and he said I would need to take a shot every day for the rest of my life. Back then, I knew very little about diabetes, but the doctor told me less than I already knew. He did say after giving me a shot that later in the evening I might feel a little funny, and if I did, I should eat something.

Following this brief encounter, I was admitted to the maternity ward . . . yes, that is correct!

That night I did indeed feel a bit unusual and obediently turned on my nurse call light. When my nurse arrived, I explained what the doctor had told me. She promptly left the room, and soon returned with two other nurses. All of them turned on every single light in the room as they hovered over my bed with panic on their faces. Sensing their fear, I simplified my request, and asked for anything they could bring me to eat.

About thirty minutes later, they proudly returned with a warm glass of milk that had been sweetened with honey. This was fitting nourishment for newborn babies, I supposed, but for me? Without a word of complaint, I gratefully drank!

The following morning, my nurse returned with a large, steel needle and proceeded to give me a shot. As she laboriously began pushing the needle along the surface of my arm, visions of a life filled with rituals of daily torture muddied my mind. With excruciating care, she slowly pierced my skin and injected some insulin. The entire process was extremely painful.

Then as quickly as it all began, I was discharged back to school with a book of exchanges telling me how many bread, vegetable, fruit, protein servings and fat I could eat at each meal, along with a roll of urine test tape. I was told to check my urine several times throughout the day, and log how many +++ signs of sugar spilled out in my urine. +1 was good, +4 less than desirable, and my insulin dosage was based on glucose levels that had changed long before the sugar spilled into my urine.

Fortunately, our school nurse knew a bit more about diabetes than those maternity ward nurses. She taught me her tricks for giving injections, showing me how to hold my syringe like a dart and pop it into my arm or leg . . . oh, how sweet the relief!

Growing up, I had not been encouraged to play sports, which might be why physical education became my greatest struggle. During softball practice, I was so weak and uncoordinated that the practice softballs often hit me right in the chest. I didn't have the energy to react or move out of the way. Because my vision was blurry, I often depended on classmates to read assignments to me. As a result, my grades suffered; at the time, I felt like I must be stupid.

Alone in a new world, among friends I barely knew, I began to cope the only way I'd ever known. I pretended as if nothing had happened, and did my best to present an appearance of effortless ease. Secretly, however, I would cry myself to sleep, wondering if I would ever feel well again, wishing it all would end. When I arrived home for the summer, I found out that my parents knew less about my diabetes than I. So life, on the surface, went on as usual.

Following graduation from Far Eastern Academy in 1979, I returned to the United States to attend a private college in Tennessee. My brother, who was already there, was pretty much a genius, and often voiced his opinion that women were intellectually inferior to men. Something in me, however, was determined to prove him wrong, so I applied myself to learning in a way I had never done in the past. By the time of our graduation, the grades from my final semester brought my GPA up to 3.76, and they actually sent my diploma back to be reprinted so it could read *magna cum laude* . . . just like my brother's!

It was around the time of my graduation from college, in May of 1983, that I received my first blood glucose meter. It was a rather bulky machine, requiring a spray of water at sixty seconds, and it took an additional sixty seconds before a reading would appear. The lancet device looked like a guillotine and hurt like one, too (not that I actually know what a guillotine feels like).

Seeing my numbers in real time made me realize that it might be a good idea to see a diabetes specialist. With considerable consternation, I made my first appointment to see an endocrinologist. I wondered what he would say about my blood sugar bouncing back and forth between 50 mg/dL and 350 mg/dL. But he said *nothing*! In fact, he told me I was doing just fine and didn't need to change a thing.

I still didn't know a lot about diabetes, but I was relatively certain that blood sugar spikes like that were not good for my body. If an endocrinologist couldn't help, what hope did I have?

In June of the same year, I married my best friend and supporter, Clyde, and began looking for a job. My Bachelor's degree in Home Economics, later embellished to the status of "Family and Consumer Economics," was already obsolete. Schools no longer hired Home Economics teachers to help students learn basic skills that could help them through life. The newspaper, however, was crowded with opportunities for nurses, and given my interest in public health, it seemed that becoming a nurse was a good idea. Clyde, who was already a nurse, helped me study to challenge first semester nursing in an effort to save money. Eighteen months later I found myself sitting for the Tennessee State Board of Nursing exam. It was during this time in nursing school that I realized my instructors knew less about diabetes than I, and the desire to help people live well with diabetes became my lifelong passion.

The first job I took as a graduate nurse was on the diabetes floor of our local hospital, but not on the end where "diabetes education" was done. Rather, I was assigned to the end where the skilled care, long term, and "ready for nursing home" patients resided. And what a *lot* of work it was. The nurses, who were already burned out, loved to assign me the most difficult patients and called me "Nancy Nurse" because I wouldn't sit down until everyone's needs were met (but quite honestly, that never happened).

Then, to add insult to injury, they chided me because they didn't think I took care of myself or my diabetes. One day, they even called one of the endocrinologists aside to ask if he thought I was taking care of myself. He abruptly asked the range of my blood glucose levels, and dutifully admonished me with a reprimand.

His comments shook me up, which is why I decided that any hope of making a good impression as a "wanna be" diabetes educator would be lost if I didn't get my blood sugar under better control before my first, upcoming appointment to see one of his colleagues. So I adjusted my insulin dosage as best I knew how. But a few weeks later (on April 17, 1986, to be exact), I found myself awakening at the scene of my own automobile accident. It was attributed to *hypoglycemia* due to the fact that I had adjusted my therapy without understanding the way insulin worked in my body. It was a moment in time that forever changed my life.

At the time of impact, my face and the steering wheel had it out, and my oral surgeon told me that repairing the damage was like trying to sew spaghetti together. As my jaw, teeth, and lower lip rotted away, and my life weighed in the balance, I reluctantly agreed to go on an insulin pump. My face was mutilated. So was my will to fight.

Self-doubt replaced my dreams. I remember thinking, Perhaps I wasn't good enough? Experiences from my past and comments from my healthcare providers left me feeling that diabetes somehow made me less of a person, and less competent than my peers in educating others about my disease. My ability to recall information on command was also affected, and I no longer felt confident in my ability to safely care for my patients. My heart felt like it had died right along with my dreams.

I flitted from job to job, hoping to find my place in the grand scheme of things; my resume soon looked like a travelogue. When I finally landed a job as a "patient educator" in a rehabilitation hospital, my hopes once again grew. But I was slighted when I applied for a job as a diabetes nurse educator in one of the local endocrinologist's offices. I thought again, *Perhaps "they" were right? Perhaps I didn't belong, and didn't have anything special to offer others who lived with my disease?*

Years later, due to a change in our insurance, it became necessary for me to find a new endocrinologist, Dr. David Huffman. When I entered Dr. Huffman's office that day, I expected more reprimands and judgments, and was primed to react. When he asked how I determined how much insulin to take for my meals, I lit into him to advise that I had to live with diabetes and had no intention of weighing and measuring my food. Sensing my anger, he quietly finished my exam, then told me that I could return whenever I liked. As he left the room with his back toward me, Dr. Huffman quietly said, "I have diabetes, too."

Finally, there was somebody who "got it!"

Talk about motivation. It was all I could do to wait another three months to come back and find out how my new endocrinologist could help.

View from the Edge

As I look back on the negativity that surrounded my relationship with diabetes and healthcare providers in my earlier years, it is surprising to note that my A1C maintained in the 4 to 5 percent range, back in the days when I didn't even know what that meant. During those years, my energy was focused on becoming "good enough." I expected far more of myself than anyone else, and as my own relentless judge, I thrived on the ability to outdo my own performance. The "high" of accomplishment was exhilarating, and it took increasingly creative feats to satisfy my addiction in order to overcome the "low" that inevitably followed in the wake of success.

I also struggled with significant disfigurement of my face and severe headaches as a result of my accident, and subsequent misalignment of my jaw. When people looked at me, they looked through me, and I often felt an urge to slap them on their face and say, "Go ahead, ask what happened." I knew that surgical osteotomy could help, but I was unable to overcome the memory of previous surgeries, the fear of "imprisonment" I'd felt while my mouth was wired shut at the time of my accident, or the belief that I somehow deserved the disfigurement.

It took several years of suffering before I succumbed and returned for eight hours of reconstructive surgery, which was indeed every bit as difficult as

I'd imagined. When the swelling subsided and my "new face" appeared, it was painful to note the difference it made in the way people responded to me. It was as if I were actually a person again.

By the time of my fortieth birthday, I'd "burned the candle at both ends" for so long that my health had declined to the point that my husband told me I was nothing more than an invalid. Sitting in a daze, I had little energy for anything outside of work and the absolute necessities of life. My diabetes and the numerous symptoms that ailed me became an obsession as I looked to discover a magical "fix" with the next tweak of a basal rate.

Yet in the midst of my struggle, I hoped once again to become the Certified Diabetes Educator (CDE) I had always believed I could be, and pay forward the kindness that was shown to me. I didn't know if my hours of work experience would qualify for the 2000 direct patient education hours that are required to write the certification exam, or if I had the physical endurance to face the daunting task of preparing for the exam. But I decided to make the commitment. I sent in my $350.00 registration fee and buckled down, determined to study one hour every day for the next six months. Flash cards, seminars, audio recordings, the CORE Curriculum for Diabetes Educators, and memorization of Clinical Practice Recommendations followed. I thought to myself, *Yes! I can* do *this!*

In May of 2001, I wrote the exam and was awarded the designation of "Certified Diabetes Educator." Afterward, I thought, *Yes! I did it!*

Earning the right to follow my name with CDE was only the beginning, however. My journey has not been easy. Yet within the seeds of discipline and desire that it took to make those first steps toward my dream was everything that was needed for the next.

Through the years as a person with diabetes, and as a diabetes educator, I have learned that most of us come to diabetes with a great deal of brokenness. This impacts our ability to live with and manage our diabetes. As women, we are schooled to believe that caring for our bodies is somehow less important than caring for everyone else. And even when we have the support of caring healthcare providers, there is a great deal of internal work we must do before we can experience true health and healing. By healing, I do not imply a cure. Healing goes much deeper than a cure, and I've come to believe that healing is far more desirable.

Hanging On to Hope

Following my auto accident in 1986, and subsequent reconstructive surgeries, the prolonged exposure to latex contributed to my development of a severe latex allergy that affects my ability to breathe, and cross-reactivity to many foods and food additives that I am no longer able to eat. My pituitary gland was also damaged, and over the years its function has progressively declined. As the "master gland of all glands," the pituitary gland tells the others what to do. I now have to replace a lot more hormones than insulin. And, as if that were not enough, I recently discovered that I also have gluten intolerance.

The complexity of all these conditions requires a great deal of time and attention on my part, and is a full time job in itself. It is necessary for me to prepare every morsel of food that I eat, and to carry that food and additional medications wherever I go. The foods that I am able to eat could be written on the palm of one hand. I have to plan for the unexpected and flex my schedule to allow recuperation after those days when I knowingly, or unexpectedly, expose myself to environmental allergens like balloons, erasers, rubber bands, a freshly vacuumed carpet, perfumes, scented candles, pollens, new blacktop paving on the highway (worse still if it's raining on freshly-laid blacktop), and much, much more. (Sometimes I have to ask for other people to help me avoid these things.) When exposed, I use inhalers, antihistamines, and extra prednisone as my body is no longer able to respond with the appropriate production of cortisol. Postural change, as I might encounter in housekeeping or other activities, can drop my blood glucose like a rock; so I have to plan. Every change in my environment, food, medication, activity, or sleep pattern requires a counterbalance in basal/ bolus insulin.

Another very personal challenge has been that of regulating my emotions. The blood glucose fluctuation of diabetes in and of itself contributes to rapid mood swings. Add to that the imbalance of multiple hormones caused by a dysfunctional pituitary gland and you have a recipe for disaster. Neural damage from my accident plays an additional role, as my brain's ability to process incoming visual stimuli is impaired. The effect is like reading through straws, with each eye working independently rather than together. My memory recall is also impaired; when trying to verbalize a word, I often describe the word I am searching for, and my friends have learned to suggest words until I say "that one!"

Lack of emotional regulation was a part of my heritage as well. As a child, expressing my anger was not tolerated, while skills for the appropriate expressions of emotion were not modeled. I reacted to life rather than responding with grace, and my inability to self-regulate cost me some of the jobs I valued most.

My quest for answers was studded with frustration and guilt, as I thought it a moral deficiency rather than a skill to be learned. Understanding my past and the way it impacts my thoughts and internal self-talk has been crucial; the development of mind-body skills that bring awareness to my body sensations, before I get to the point of explosion, has been key. Exercise, yoga, and

33

mindfulness are now essential components of the balance I seek, and it has taken a great deal of "not knowing" to discover what works for me.

Not knowing can be extremely uncomfortable and incapacitating. It can lead to considerable "*dis*-ease" and "*dis*-stress" as your mind goes in multiple directions trying to determine what will happen next. In so doing, it is easy to miss what is happening in the present moment, which is indeed the only moment that is ours to live.

In my search for answers, I discovered the incredible power of our minds in determining the outcome of our lives, and the incredible joy of living in the present moment. Learning to live in the "now" has helped me develop a keener awareness and understanding of my body and its needs, and brings meaning in the midst of my chaos. So, as strange as this may sound, I find that gratitude towards my diabetes and the numerous other physical challenges I face has helped me to develop the courage and skills necessary to transcend my physical limitations and become more than I could otherwise have been.

Jumping Again

Turning fifty was a big deal for me, and it was a milestone I am proud to announce! I don't know that I ever consciously thought about it, but somewhere in the back of my mind, there was a belief that I would not live very long because I had diabetes. The first time I met someone who had lived with diabetes for more than thirty years, it was an unexpected surprise. Now, having lived with diabetes for more than thirty-three years myself, it is pleasing to note that I have no complications from the disease. I now know that it is very possible to live a long and healthy life with diabetes. Through trial and error, persistence, and the help of a dedicated endocrinologist, I am generally able to maintain my A1C between 6 and 6.5 percent without undue risk of severe *hypoglycemia*.

I have found that making a difference in the lives of others is the only thing that brings meaning. Asking myself, "Will my choices today make a difference for someone ten years from now?" helps to put things in perspective on those days when life is full and things do not go as planned. My daily choice to live with optimism once prompted a friend to query if I ever experienced a "low" moment. And my quick, emphatic response was, "Absolutely . . . numerous times, every single day . . . but a positive attitude beats the alternative, and the choice is mine."

In my years of work as a CDE, I have thoroughly enjoyed my roles as a Diabetes Educator, Clinical Research Coordinator, and Certified Pump Trainer. I have a curious mind, and continually push my limits by observing, exploring, and trying new things.

When dLife asked me to help with their "Ask an Expert" Q&A back in 2006, stepping out of my traditional role as a diabetes educator was a bit unnerving. Learning how to use technology has been a challenge, as I never dreamed there would be a need to set up a Website and learn how to edit. It took months for me to build up the courage to set up a Facebook account, and Twitter . . . now, *that* was downright scary. Yet I've done it because there is need for diabetes educators to step out of the box and stretch the boundaries of the way things have always been done. Our world is changing and our work becomes obsolete if we fail to change with it.

I have learned that our experiences in life are never wasted unless we so choose; and as an outgrowth of my diverse and assorted skills and experience, my dreams have grown. Through persistence and commitment, those dreams have become reality in a bigger and better way than I ever thought possible.

Working with a group of like-minded individuals, who live as I do with diabetes, we have established a non-profit organization to provide a place where people with diabetes can come for inspiration, information, and support. As Program Coordinator for *Partners & Peers for Diabetes Care, Inc.*, it is my pleasure to help develop both online and community programs, educational materials, and technologies that support people along their journey with diabetes. I am also training to become a certified health coach, and helping to pilot a diabetes health coaching program with use of video remote technologies.

Is living life on the edge unnerving? Often . . . but I choose, yet again, to jump!

Website: www.partnersandpeers.org

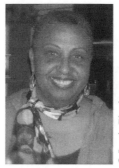

© Louis Ebarb

Chapter 4 *by Lorraine Brooks, MPH, CEAP*

From Anger to Acceptance

This chapter is dedicated to my mother, Ida, who passed away earlier this year as I was writing this chapter, and never knew I was involved in this project. I wanted to surprise her by letting her read this chapter in book form, rather than in draft form, but that was not meant to be. I can only say I miss her dearly, and I hope that my words will mean as much to others as they would have meant to her.

My story, on the surface, is pretty much like anyone else's. When I found out I had diabetes I was surprised, but not shocked; disappointed, but not overwhelmed. My paternal grandmother had it, so I knew it ran in the family. I had seen my father give my grandmother insulin injections since I was a young child, so even that didn't seem foreign or scary.

I was diagnosed in 1984, during a routine examination for a new job in a hospital. I was immediately referred to an endocrinologist on staff, and thus, without much fanfare, I began my relationship with this disease. My fasting blood sugar was 180 mg/dL on that routine blood test. I was 32 years old, overweight (as I had been for most of my life), and I had never had any of the classic signs or symptoms of diabetes.

Although it was in my immediate family, I really did not understand how diabetes worked, what it really meant, or how it could affect my life, other than daily injections. I was put on an insulin regimen right away, without even a discussion about pills or other options. I was, of course, admonished to lose weight and follow a 1200-calorie diet, but that seemed, to me, like a no-brainer, even if I didn't have diabetes. I had been hearing that all my life!

Fortunately, I worked in the pharmacy department of the hospital, and the staff there was wonderful in their support of me and my new diagnosis. The chief pharmacist explained all about the mechanics of the disease, about insulin, and how to prepare and give myself injections. They took excellent care of me. Even the drug company sales representatives brought me alcohol swabs, lancets, and other supplies to get me started with testing.

It was all so matter-of-fact, that I didn't have time to absorb how I felt about it. I was taken care of, encouraged, and understood. I was told that this was by no means a death sentence or even a hardship, and that if I took good care of myself, I would be okay. My workmates explained that this is a disease that can certainly be controlled, and good control would mean no complications, or at least fewer complications. I had everything and everyone I needed at my disposal. On one hand I felt lucky and protected, and I was reluctant to feel anything other than grateful. But on the inside, I felt something other than gratitude.

I would not be telling the truth if I didn't say how angry I was, and in some ways still am, that I have diabetes. My journey with this disease has been, in reality, an angry one, but it has also been one of hope and courage and acceptance. It first began with anger, because pretty soon after the diagnosis, I began to realize how much the necessary self-care was going to intrude on my active lifestyle, though I had no idea how much I would come to depend on my blood glucose meter. I also didn't know that "numbers" would begin to play such an important role. My parents were alive and well, and there was no real illness or disability in my family. My grandmother's diabetes was a distant memory.

The real anger set in when I realized that I needed to begin paying attention to things and situations that, at one time, I could do without any thought at all. I soon learned that diabetes is not just about "sugar," but is a constellation of seemingly unrelated pieces that all work together to cause the body to respond in certain ways. (It was an eye-opener, to say the least.) Not only did I have to be careful *what* I ate, but when and how much. And the "when" and "how much" were as important as the "what". At times, the "when" was the *most* important. I had never thought about any of these things before.

In my then-naïve mind, insulin was just another drug; if I took it as directed, it would simply do what it was supposed to do. I thought of it like a blood pressure medication. In other words, once I took the medication, it would "work," and I needn't do anything else. I thought that taking the insulin would control this disease with little input from me. I soon found out how wrong I was.

One of the first times I took insulin, I had a low blood sugar reaction but I didn't know what was happening. I realize it now, but at the time, I didn't know that I needed to do anything. Now, I would rush to get my meter and take a reading, but then, I just rode it out, sort of waiting to feel better. I had no idea that might be dangerous!

Looking back, I can see that in many ways the diagnosis of diabetes forced me to come to grips not only with the diagnosis itself, but with *life*. It was obvious that I needed to make changes, but I didn't know where to begin.

The most obvious needed change was with regards to my weight. I had struggled with my weight for as long as I could remember, seemingly since birth. Some articles I read claimed that losing weight could actually enable a person to reduce, or even eliminate, the need for diabetes medications. After reading that, I was "in." Suddenly, I didn't want any part of this disease; anything I could do to get rid of it was fine with me.

I dieted with a vengeance. And sure enough, I was able to lose five dress sizes in less than a year. And, also, just as the articles had said, I no longer needed insulin injections. In fact, I didn't need any medication at all!

I was able to control the diabetes with diet and exercise for many years. I was in a "honeymoon phase." I call it a *honeymoon*, because it felt good, and new, and important, and like it would last forever. While I was in this honeymoon period, I finished my undergraduate degree, got my first real career-oriented job, and it seemed like the world was my oyster. I was in a good relationship, happy in my circle of friends, and had the respect of everyone around me. So it goes when you are taking good care of yourself and people can see results.

The problem I found is that with this disease, even the best self-care sometimes isn't enough. Add in the weight-loss battle to the mix and you have two life-long fights, with varying degrees of success along the way. So that is where I try to stay in my emotional battle – that is, to remind myself that I will have good days and bad days, that some of it is out of my control, and that like anything else in life, there will be times when no effort will yield success – times when even the most monumental effort will fall short.

I did my best to hold onto this attitude when I decided to go back to school for a Master's degree. I had been working full-time as the Director of an Employee Assistance Program at a major medical center, teaching part-time at Brooklyn College, taking care of elderly relatives, and was in a not-so-satisfying relationship. At the time, I felt like I needed to make some changes, and none of those situations were "changeable" in the ways I needed. Going to graduate school was something I had always wanted to do, but I had made some decisions that initially carried my life in a different direction. But I knew I would do it eventually – and 2001 turned out to be the "eventually" I had been waiting for.

With a great deal of trepidation, I began my coursework. I started off very slowly – with one course per semester – because I still had all those other things on my plate. I also decided to become a New York City Auxiliary Policewoman that same year. So I had a full-time job, a part-time job, caretaking, training for

NYPD Auxiliary, and graduate school on my plate at the same time. And, oh, yes, I also continued managing my diabetes. This was during the honeymoon phase, where I was able to get by with diet and exercise alone, so I didn't have to worry about injections and low blood sugar. But it was still difficult and stressful.

My life fell apart at least three times during the six years it took to get my Master's degree.

First, there was September 11, 2001. I had just finished my Auxiliary training, and hadn't even been issued a badge or uniform when the attacks occurred. I had completed my training and taken the test in August, receiving the highest mark among the graduates of that training program. I was all ready to be sworn in and get the vouchers for uniforms and supplies when the planes hit the World Trade Center. Suddenly, protocol was unimportant, and it was all-hands-on-deck. Including auxiliaries.

With a borrowed uniform I swung into action. School was suspended in NYC as were many regular activities, so I was able to devote time to NYPD activities. It was hard to be on patrol, sometimes for hours at a time, standing, in full uniform, without eating or knowing when I would be able to eat. Not being on insulin at that time proved to be a true blessing, because it enabled me to work long hours in service to the City with minimal disruption to my health. I carried my glucose meter and granola bars in my uniform pockets.

The second thing that happened was that my dear and favorite aunt passed away in early 2003, after she'd spent over a month in hospice. It was a long battle for both of us, with some difficult decisions along the way. Up to that point, saying "no" to life-support for her had been the most difficult thing I had ever done. She had no children, and she left me in charge of probating her estate, which meant selling her home (a home I had basically grown up in) and disposing of her belongings. Many nights, after working all day and going to class, I would go to her house to pack up her things, and get the house ready for sale.

In the mornings I would pack two full meals and a few snacks, because I knew I would not be home until very late. Often, though, I ended up eating in the company cafeteria for lunch, grabbing something fast and handy before teaching, and then buying take-out on the way to my aunt's house at nine o'clock at night. This was not the best regimen for diabetes control, and I sometimes wondered why I was okay. As always, I tested my blood sugar many times a day (five or more), so I knew I was not in danger.

I became proficient at analyzing fast-food menus quickly. I tried to make healthy choices and most of the time I succeeded, but not always. I found out that salads are not always the lowest calorie or lowest fat choices! (That is a piece of information that I have used many times since.) It was during this time that I really learned to read menus, and count carbohydrates.

I could feel that I was turning some kind of corner. I was now in my fifties, and I felt that I would not be able to maintain this schedule and lifestyle too much longer on diet and exercise alone. And sure enough, not long after, I was told that I needed to begin insulin injections again. The "honeymoon" had actually lasted almost eight years. Fortunately, it wasn't a big shock, and I was able to resume insulin injections with relatively little adjustment.

I should mention that one of the drug company's representatives told me about insulin pens. I was intrigued with the idea of not having to stop what I was doing in order to take a shot of insulin. (Before eating, I would usually excuse myself and go to a bathroom to give myself a shot in privacy.) I spoke to my doctor, and he agreed to let me switch from syringes, where I had to withdraw the dose and fill it myself, to the new pre-filled insulin pens. Since I used both a long-acting and short-acting insulin, I needed two separate pens.

This change turned out to be a good one because I could take a shot, without having to excuse myself, and that suited me well. Many times, before teaching, I could take my shot while the students were filing into the room, or even while doing the preliminaries for the lesson; it was that easy.

Many times I would even tell the students what I was doing and we would talk about it. Since I taught classes in health education, I made it part of the class discussion and used myself as an example. I don't know if this was a good "by the book" teaching method, but I know it was effective because often, at the end of the semester, students would tell me that my honesty and openness was helpful to them. Some had friends with diabetes, and my examples helped them to understand what they were dealing with. Some students had diabetes in their families and they were encouraged to take better care of themselves.

The next big thing that disrupted my life happened on December 21, 2004, when my best friend died, unexpectedly, after surgery. We'd had a conversation before she went into the hospital about arrangements, etc., the sort of conversation you *have to have* so that "just in case" anything happens, you will know what to do. I wasn't the least bit interested in having that conversation – after all she was only fifty-two years old, and the procedure was relatively common – but as a courtesy I listened, agreeing that if anything "happened," I would do exactly as she wanted and tucked away all of the information.

When the phone rang, I felt as if I had been hit by a train. The call came while I was at my full-time job and was ready to see a client. I saw the client, told him what had just happened, and apologized for having to test my blood sugar in front of him. He was very understanding and offered to come at another time. But he had made a long trip to see me for counseling and I thought I was okay enough to go ahead.

41

I must have swung into automatic pilot as one does when extremely stressful things happen, and I really don't remember much about that moment except thinking, *I need to test my blood sugar because I think I'm going to pass out.* Somehow, my diabetes instinct kicked in even before anything else, because above all I wanted and needed to make sure I was okay before I did anything, or especially before I went anywhere (driving).

After he left, I vaguely remember packing up my bag. I did my best to take everything I would need "just in case" I didn't go to work for a few days. The first things I made sure I had were my insulin pens and my glucose meter. Even in the face of personal tragedy, my priority was to take care of myself. I still sometimes marvel at this, but I have come to realize that when things get tough, it is even *more* important for me to practice good self-care.

I planned a memorial service for my friend, did all the things she asked me to do, and I was strong during the whole ordeal. I kept my blood sugar in check by doing what I had learned to do – namely, test my blood sugar several times a day, eat less rather than more, make sure I got to bed early, and focused on my emotional needs as well as physical ones.

As I got up to do her eulogy at the service (as I had promised her I would), I felt weak. Did I feel weak because of my blood sugar, or because of what I was about to do? Not knowing, I made my usual announcement that while I was speaking, I needed to check my blood sugar. No one batted an eyelash, and once again I learned the lesson that for me, honesty was the best policy. I could see the faces in the church waiting to get a sign from me that I needed juice or a snack, but I was okay. I continued on.

What these events have in common is that they were life-altering. I described them earlier as "my life fell apart," and that is exactly what happened (in different ways). All three events were unexpected, and all of them had a profound effect on me emotionally as well as physically.

If having diabetes can ever be considered a blessing, I can see it in the fact that during each of these events, I still managed to take care of myself *because I had to.* And I emphasize that phrase because I don't know if I would have taken the same care of myself if I didn't *have to.*

The overarching sentiment for me is, "diabetes first, anything else after." Just as they tell you on airplanes or cruise ships that you should save yourself first, that is what you *must* do with diabetes. Save yourself first; then you can save or help others. For me, diabetes has been that "saving myself first" mantra. No matter what happens, diabetes has to be my priority.

It hasn't all been a walk in the park. A few years ago, I began to notice that my blood sugar was getting higher and higher, regardless of what I did to keep it down. The regimens that I used to follow were no longer effective.

Up until this point, I had been an exercise buff. Riding twenty minutes a day on a stationary bicycle was enough to keep my glucose in check for many years. I could even indulge in extra carbohydrates and get away with it, if I was willing to ride an extra five or ten minutes. All of a sudden, riding the bike was having little or no effect on my blood sugar control. Around this time, I went back to Weight Watchers®, because I noticed my weight creeping up as well.

Nothing seemed to be working. I was doing twice the work, with less than half the results. I was getting very frustrated and worried. I explained the situation to my doctor, but he wasn't interested in hearing my story. He admonished me to lose weight (but didn't tell me how), and told me that this was just "something I had to accept about aging and having diabetes."

His comments did not sit well with me. By this time, I had lived with diabetes for almost twenty-five years. I knew what to do, and how my body responded to my regimen.

But the problem wasn't me, or what I wasn't doing right. The problem was diabetes. (So, my doctor may have been right about that.) There is a progression to the disease, and in spite of doing all the "right" things, sometimes things change, and the changes are beyond our control. We have to adjust to them.

At this point, I think my anger fueled me to do something which turned out to be one of the best things I have done in relation to having diabetes. I sought the help of a new doctor and began to ask some difficult questions. And I started using an insulin pump.

Because I knew that I needed some new input, I found an endocrinologist and have worked with her for the past three years. My previous doctor was a general practitioner, and although he was good in many ways, I didn't feel he understood my experiences.

As for deciding to use the insulin pump, I had heard about this option from a friend who is a nurse. I had no idea what to expect or how insulin pumps worked, but I was willing to give it a try as I kind of enjoy being on the cutting edge. I'm fortunate that I have access to such things, and I am lucky to have very good health insurance coverage, which I know is a blessing.

There probably isn't an easy way to deal with diabetes, but with my pump, the one thing I don't have to worry about is injections. The pump provides a constant basal infusion, and when I eat, I can calculate the amount of carbohydrates and give myself a bolus dose to cover what I am eating. It doesn't require privacy in the same way that I needed when I would give myself injections. (I remember going out to lunch on a "first date" with someone, and having to ask them if they minded watching me give myself an injection. At least I don't need to do that any more.)

I realize now that one of the issues I had with having diabetes was that I felt like it was public, and I didn't want it to be. I didn't want it to be known to people who were not necessarily in my circle, because in my experience, I have found that some people tend to judge and make assumptions about people with diabetes. I do not handle people like that very well, as I tend to be a private person, and I do not like receiving unsolicited advice about how to handle my illness. I found that having an insulin pump has eliminated some of that feeling because I no longer have to take time or excuse myself to prepare an injection. It is still sometimes a topic of conversation, but in ways I find less intrusive.

Insulin pumps are not for everyone. There is a lot of time and attention involved, but I find it easier to use than syringes or pens. I also find that since it is easier for me, my glucose control is better than it had been. I still test myself several times a day, and of course I still have to be mindful of what, when, and how much I eat, and when I exercise, etc. The insulin pump doesn't make diabetes any easier, but for me it certainly has made diabetes management easier.

The most recent chapter in my journey happened very recently. As I write this, it has been about six weeks since I lost my dear mother. She died on her ninety-sixth birthday. I have to say it was sudden and shocking, even though she was at an advanced age. My mother must have wondered how much time she could possibly have left, and I could sense that she was just plain tired. In the end, we sat and watched TV (especially her beloved baseball team, the Mets!), and we talked about life. We both knew her days were numbered, but we never mentioned that. We simply enjoyed each other's company.

My mother did not have diabetes. She could eat and drink anything she wanted, and I was always a little jealous of that. She'd have bacon and eggs every morning, and until the last year or so, she had a cocktail each night with her dinner. She used real butter, ate white bread and pasta, never exercised, never had a weight problem, and loved anything sweet – the joke in my family always was how my mother would only eat dinner so she could eat dessert. It was always amazing to me the differences in our eating habits. (She was never a particularly good cook, either, as many mothers are.) I would think to myself, *if I ate those things, I would be 300 pounds!*

Bless her heart, she never really got the hang of *why* I need to eat the way I do. I think she was someone who assumed that diabetes is all about sugar, and as long as you avoided sugar you would be all right. Of course, I only wish that were true. Our pantry was always filled with at least two kinds of everything you can imagine – white rice for her, brown rice for me; whole milk for her, skim milk for me; butter for her, light margarine for me; sugar for her, sugar substitute for me; white bread for her, whole wheat bread for me; ice cream for her, fat-free, no sugar added frozen yogurt for me. The list goes on and on.

When I went grocery shopping last week for the first time to buy groceries for just *me*, it was difficult to make choices, as silly as that sounds. I found myself reaching for all of those old items, and reminding myself that I no longer have to buy them. It was a bittersweet feeling.

I have now begun the task of discarding all the food items that I know I will not use. This is also bittersweet, but necessary. I will now stock my kitchen with only the things I need and enjoy.

Living alone is also going to be different in another way. I don't think my mother understood that when my blood sugar was low or going down fast that I needed to eat or drink something right away. That was actually a source of frustration, living with someone who didn't understand the way this disease works. This is sometimes a lonely journey.

It will be an interesting ride from this point forward. I will have to readjust to being single, older, a little more fragile, and continuing to cope with a chronic illness that can take a lot of time and energy to control. The good news for me is that I am both attentive and vigilant, so not much gets past me. I now have an endocrinologist who listens, pays attention, and is willing to work with me. She does not lecture me; instead, she takes the time to explain, in my terms, what is happening.

I believe this is half the battle, as you have to find a doctor and other healthcare professionals with whom you can work, and with whom you can be totally honest. We are not perfect, and we will have days, weeks, or even months maybe, where we will fall "off the wagon" in terms of being diligent. The worst thing that can happen is for my doctor to treat me in a manner that makes me feel as if I am a bad child who did not obey the rules. Some of my friends have physicians who treat them that way, and I can see that it actually makes them *less* compliant and even more frustrated.

Today I choose to honor myself, with all my flaws, and all my shortcomings, and all my inconsistencies. I know I am not perfect, but I strive to be the best I can be at any given moment, and to make the best decisions I can make with the information I have. And I forgive myself for making not-so-healthy choices on occasion, because I'm allowed to make mistakes.

All in all, I have to say it has been a positive journey. The one thing that is a constant is that I keep learning about myself in this process. Every day poses new challenges, and I have to continue to adjust in order to stay healthy and safe. I have learned not just about my body, but about my emotional self as well. My reactions, responses, feelings, and perspectives have become more important to me because of having diabetes.

I have had to make myself *the* priority, for all aspects of life. For example, I have learned how to respond to people who sometimes make insensitive comments. I used to get frustrated, even angry, and I am sure I overreacted at times, which may have pushed some people away due to my responses. But I believe time and experience have mellowed me, and I can now deal with people differently.

If I had the opportunity to say anything to people without diabetes, I would say a few things about how to treat me.

First, don't be the "food police." Usually, people with diabetes know exactly what we are doing, and we know it may look wrong to *you*, but that doesn't necessarily mean it is "wrong." While we have to maintain a delicate balance, that doesn't mean we can't eat ice cream or an occasional small slice of cake.

Second, don't feel sorry for me. I don't want pity.

Third, please don't offer unsolicited advice. Sometimes, people who don't have diabetes don't understand the issues we face daily, and may be quick to judge. Support is great, and we need it. And useful information is always welcome.

So far, after almost thirty years with diabetes, I have not experienced any complications. I knock wood as I write this, but I also believe that it is in no small part because I try to take excellent care of myself. I eat a balanced diet, get regular exercise, and I see my healthcare professionals regularly. Those are the most important things I can do.

In recent months, I have revisited an interest I had years ago. I have begun to write again. I write poetry, prose, and short stories, and I have even begun to work on my autobiography, "Sweet Lorraine." I find that writing is not only fun and interesting, but it is also therapeutic. I'm proud to have my poem, entitled "My Sweet Life," serve as the Prologue to this book.

I used to believe that no one would be interested in anything I had to say, but I now know that is not true. We all have wisdom to share, and as we travel this particular journey with diabetes, I think we can use all the wisdom we can get! I also used to believe that I was alone in my struggles, and that my experiences were unique. I used to blame myself for having "bad" days, or making "bad" choices. I do that a lot less now. Today I embrace my humanity, and I honor my voice. And most of all, I consider myself lucky to live a sweet life.

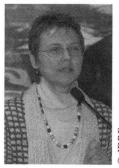

Chapter 5   *by Carol Grafford, RD, CDE*

Enemy, Neighbor, Dancer, Teacher

The Beginning

How do you begin the story of your life? I believe in the river of life, where each of us is a continuation of our parents and grandparents, our ancestors. To say who you are, you have to say something about those who came before you.

I feel that I was born into the luckiest of circumstances, as I received great gifts from both parents.

My mother was (and still is) competent, confident, capable and creative. My mother was firm and strong; she believed in hard work. From my mom I received the gift of believing in myself, as I knew that I could be or do anything to which I set my mind.

My father was kind, quiet, forgiving, accepting, tolerant and flexible. My father was curious, a thinker, a lover of history, philosophy and sociology; he believed in education. From my dad, I received the gifts of broad-thinking, flexibility and compassion; I also learned how to listen well and to speak diplomatically. In other words, not only could I accomplish anything I wanted (reinforcing my mother's gift), I could also do things in a way that helped people rather than hurt them.

I grew up in the rural Midwest, in southwestern Michigan. My childhood felt happy, safe and secure. My parents always believed that we were poor, but my sisters and I didn't share that sentiment. My dad believed that books were wonderful, but he also believed that if you could see an elephant in the zoo, that would be a better education that just reading about elephants in a book.

So we traveled a lot. Car trips to Florida mostly, to visit grandparents who lived there. And every car trip was "an adventure" – whether we stopped at a historical marker along the road, or had a flat tire in the mountains of Kentucky – everything we did was adventurous.

In the summer of 1975, between my junior and senior years of high school, I had my biggest travel adventure yet – I was accepted as an exchange student to the Philippines! I lived for two months with a middle class family in a suburb of Manila. We had many adventures in the big city, but also took several trips to "the provinces" – i.e., the rural areas. I loved the people, their language, the warm ocean, the water buffaloes, and the rice paddies terraced into the mountains. It was a wonderful and exotic experience.

Then I started losing weight. I had been tall and thin my whole life, so I didn't need to lose any weight. When I flew to the Philippines, I was 5 feet 8 inches tall and weighed 118 pounds – my height, blonde hair and fair skin made me stick out like a sore thumb. Now, six weeks after I'd flown over, I was losing weight and drinking about two liters of beverages at each meal.

At first, this didn't bother me. I thought, Of *course I'm thirsty – it's hot here!* And because I was an American teen, I wasn't worried about getting thinner – didn't everybody want that? But I was bothered by cramps in my legs at night, and when they woke me up, I would always have to urinate; I thought the cramps were far worse than having to run to the bathroom. A local doctor prescribed B-complex vitamins for the leg cramps, and they did seem to help.

After a while, my "foster mom" in Manila asked me for a urine sample. She took it to her friends at Santo Thomas, the local teaching hospital. The results came back while I was visiting a Filipino friend in another part of town. My "foster mom" was so concerned, she sent a taxi to pick me up immediately. I was taken directly to Santo Thomas.

I was told that there was no question. I had diabetes.

I will never forget that taxi ride, as I spent the whole ride sobbing and crying. I said things like "Why me?!" and "It can't be true!"

Once at the hospital, I remember being in a small, private room with short, young Filipino nurses coming to see me in groups of about six or so at a time. They were all between four and five feet tall, and wore crisp white dresses – the old-fashioned nursing uniform, along with those archaic white nurse's caps. By this time, I had lost twenty pounds – yes, I really was a ninety-eight-pound weakling! (My few photos from the hospital show me as a long-haired skeleton with skin – pretty scary.)

The student nurses taught me to inject insulin. I wasn't scared – my mother had taught me that I could do anything. And I was highly motivated to do whatever the doctors said was important. But to fully understand my motivation, you have to go farther back in my family.

50

In 1943, when my mother was only five years old, her mother gave birth to a stillborn son. It was the second time she'd lost a child this way, but now they understood the reason: diabetes. Soon, diabetes became a "normal" part of my mother's childhood. Since my own family spent a whole day at grandma's house every week, diabetes was a "normal" part of my childhood, too.

Grandma was in many ways defined by her diabetes. But to my sisters and me, she was a mean old lady who complained a lot (mostly about her health), and kept a candy dish in every room of her house. She also had three cookie jars and a whole drawer full of candy in the kitchen. Our grandpa ate cookies every day, and we could usually get permission for a cookie or two, but the candy drawer was forbidden to us kids. Of course, we peeked in there often and it was always full, but never with the same items.

By the time I was a teen, I had seen my grandma sneak hundreds of pieces of candy from the candy dishes and the secret drawer. At the same time, grandma's trips to the hospital became more and more frequent – it was always something to do with her diabetes. I knew that the grown-ups were worried that grandma might die this time. Because of this, I judged my grandma harshly over the way she cared for her diabetes. My opinion of her was not very high.

So there I was, seventeen years old, a patient in Santo Thomas, the university hospital in Manila, Philippines. I'd gotten over the "Why me?" feeling pretty quickly, and vowed that I would be absolutely nothing like my grandmother! I would do everything *perfectly* – follow the diet, take the injections, do whatever they told me to do.

This vow was strongly reinforced shortly after I flew back home. When I got there, grandma was yet again in the hospital. By now, she had every full-blown complication of diabetes in the medical books: blindness, kidney disease, heart disease, nerve damage and the inability to heal.

She had become blind due to retinal hemorrhages long before I'd gone to the Philippines. Now, she had late-stage kidney failure as well, because Grandma's kidneys could no longer remove any waste or excess water from her blood. Her legs became so swollen with fluid that her skin would "weep" salt water. Since the excess fluids have nowhere to go, they build up in the body tissues, especially in the lungs and the legs. This made it hard for grandma to breathe.

Some people think you would feel sad or overwhelmed at seeing your grandmother this way, and maybe part of me felt those things. But what I remember the most was feeling angry – angry that grandma did this to herself and angry that she seemed to create so much drama and suffering for her family. It was as if she was manipulating them with her self-induced health problems.

Two months after I got home, several of grandma's toes had become gangrenous. The doctors were scheduled to amputate her dead toes the next day, but grandma died during the night. When the autopsy was done, they found heart and coronary artery disease so severe that even though grandma was only fifty-six years old, the inside of her body was like that of a ninety-eight year old.

All of this is why at only seventeen years of age, I had vowed, "I will do everything perfectly for my diabetes, and these bad things will not happen to me." Grandma had served as an excellent negative role model.

Scary Times

I suppose the birth of my children should have been scary, but I was blissfully undereducated at the time and didn't know enough to be scared.

My first child was born in 1979 in Michigan's rural Upper Peninsula (the UP), with the nearest obstetrician over 100 miles away. Worse than that, the nearest diabetes specialist was 500 miles away. Jenny was born three weeks early, but we were lucky; after a week or so in the hospital, she was fine.

My second child was born in 1982 in metropolitan Minneapolis. My family doctor there referred me to an obstetrician who specialized in high-risk pregnancies – supposedly, anyway. I found that he actually provided much less care than my family practice doctor in the UP. This new doctor had me "come back in three months," where I had been seen weekly the first time. But I was ignorant, and figured he must know what he was doing. It was the obstetrician's nurse who clued me in on blood glucose meters. She helped with my insurance, and taught me how to use my first-ever blood glucose meter, but by then I was seven months along!

Kate was born on time and healthy, but she was very big at birth – almost eleven pounds. Neither doctor had ever referred me to a dietitian or a diabetes educator for either pregnancy – yikes!

Before, during, and after my pregnancies, I was happily going along, doing all the things the doctors wanted, "perfectly." That is to say, whatever they told me to do, I did. I followed the diet. I took the insulin. I tested my urine and my blood.

One night, my husband, Jim, and I ate popcorn for our bedtime snack. In my old diet books, two cups of popcorn was one exchange. I measured exactly, as I always did. I had already taken my insulin at supper like I was supposed to, and I ate exactly the amount of carbohydrate I was supposed to.

That night, around 2:00 AM, I suffered a *grand mal* seizure due to *hypoglycemia* (low blood sugar). Jim called 9-1-1, and tried to treat my low blood sugar by smearing pancake syrup inside my cheeks. He had to call a neighbor to watch our two small girls. I woke up in the hospital emergency room several hours later.

That was the scariest experience of my life. I was twenty-six years old and realized for the first time that diabetes could kill me even if I did everything "perfectly."

I took steps to make sure this wouldn't happen again. I called the American Diabetes Association (ADA) and asked for help. They referred me to the support group in my local area that was run by a wonderful woman named Barbara Keller. She was a RN, BSN, and also one of the first people ever credentialed as a Certified Diabetes Educator (CDE).

The support group was wonderful and helped me immensely. There, I first learned about *glucagon* – the emergency injection for severe *hypoglycemia*. After nine years with type 1 diabetes, I had never heard of *glucagon* before! I also learned how to find a diabetes specialist. He helped me drop my A1C value from 9 percent to 7 percent. But the most important thing I gained from the support group was a mentor, as I saw how much Barbara Keller helped people with diabetes. She herself didn't have diabetes, but that didn't matter; she was kind and gentle and knowledgeable. I thought: *When I grow up (ha ha!) I want to be just like her.*

Success

Success is defined in many ways. One of my favorite definitions is from Deepak Chopra: "The continued expansion of happiness and the progressive realization of worthy goals." Maybe the reason I like this definition so much is because the key word here is *goals*.

When I was a little kid, my dad's employer had given him a yellow sticker that was about five inches square. It read. "What will you do to reach your moon today?" (It was kind of silly.) This was just after the 1969 moon launch, when humans first walked on the moon. Dad put the sticker on the kitchen cabinet near the refrigerator, and it stayed there until long after I moved away from home. You couldn't miss that bright yellow reminder.

Goal-setting was natural in our house. I remember when I was about sixteen (before the diabetes struck) that I thought about my life goals. I decided there were three important ones: to get a college education, to raise a family, and to own my own home.

By the time I was thirty, I was married, with children, and we owned our own home (although there was a mortgage involved!) I was a full-time homemaker at the time, and happy. But I felt that if I didn't get my college degree soon, I would never get around to it. That's when I went back to school.

I did some research trying to decide how I could follow in my mentor's footsteps. I learned that to be a CDE at that time, you must be a medical doctor, a registered nurse, or a registered dietitian before you could even think about working toward the CDE. I decided that becoming a registered dietitian was my best route.

I started with just one class at the local community college, but soon was going full-time. After two years, I was accepted into the Coordinated Program in Nutrition and Dietetics at the University of Minnesota. It was a tough program that jammed all the usual requirements for lectures, labs and exams that you need for a BS degree, plus a 1000 hour internship in dietetics, all into the last two years of college.

The internship exposed me to a wide variety of employment opportunities. I got experience in everything from day cares and health spas to hospitals and nursing homes. One of the internship experiences was a week-long professional education course held at the International Diabetes Center. In another, I was sent to a hospital where a registered dietitian was running a diabetes education program that was recognized by the American Diabetes Association (ADA). (This gave me a new goal, something to add to both my career and life goals list. Now, I knew that I wanted to run an ADA-recognized diabetes education program in the rural Midwest, ideally in Michigan's Upper Peninsula.) At age thirty-six, I had my BS degree in Nutrition – another of my original life goals met – and now was ready to reach for a new goal.

Six months after I had my college diploma, I took and passed the national registration exam for dietitians – I was now a Registered Dietitian (RD)! I worked in the Minneapolis area for about a year as a nutrition educator for a set of three medical clinics owned by a group of physicians. It wasn't my dream job, but it was a great start – I was helping people who had various problems involving food: infant feeding problems, bowel disorders, obesity, high cholesterol, and yes, diabetes.

When my husband lost his job in Minneapolis due to downsizing, we stumbled on a great job opportunity for *me* – a clinical dietitian job at the local hospital back in the area we loved, Michigan's Upper Peninsula (the UP). This also wasn't my dream job, but it *was* our dream location, which is why we uprooted our family and moved. As it turned out, the job was pretty good, too.

When you live in a small rural area, if you are a dietitian, you do *all* the dietitian jobs. I worked with hospital patients, nursing home residents, outpatients (like my first job), and community outreach. I enjoyed the variety, and was still helping people, many of whom had diabetes.

When my new boss, also a RD, learned of my interest in diabetes education, she decided it was high time her hospital provided that service. She felt that ADA recognition was too expensive, but certification by the State of

Michigan was within our reach. Together, we put together a program and started offering classes. Our program was certified in 1997 – two years after I moved my family to the UP.

While all this was going on, the regional dietetic association was coming to a close due to a lack of volunteer leadership. Both my boss and I felt that our professional group was too important to dissolve, so we volunteered. She became the President, and I was President-Elect of our fifteen-county region. While my boss did not stay involved in our professional board of directors, I never left.

From the regional association, I proceeded to join the state board of directors at the Michigan Dietetic Association (MDA). I served in various positions over time, including becoming its President for 2002 to 2003.

In my paid job, after three years as a clinical dietitian, I switched to a position as community health educator. I still helped many people through support groups, wellness programs, and occasionally taught a diabetes class, but I was seeing fewer people with diabetes. The diabetes education program was still in place, but other staff members were running it and seeing the diabetes patients.

In 2001, when my boss moved out of the area, the hospital re-structured. I was given the job of Diabetes Coordinator – a full-time job that would coordinate all of the diabetes activities for the hospital. Finally, my dream job had arrived!

Within six months, I passed the exam to follow in my mentor's footsteps and became a Certified Diabetes Educator. Our diabetes education program was ADA recognized as well as state certified – which meant that this career goal had also been met!

When my term was up as MDA President in 2003, I was asked to serve on the board of the regional association of diabetes educators. Once again, I went from the regional board to the state level, this time with the Michigan Organization of Diabetes Educators (MODE). I continued to serve in various capacities, including President, until 2010.

I remember giving a speech in college around age thirty. At the time, I thought that without modern medicine, no one in the classroom would have heard my speech because I would have died at age seventeen. If that had happened, I wouldn't have married or had any children to love, nurture and watch as they grew up. My life would have just ended.

Around that time, I started to think that if I could help just one person with diabetes – *really* help them – that I would have paid back the wonderful gift of life modern medicine had given me. Through my career choices, I have been able to help many hundreds of people. And maybe I have even been able to *really* help a small handful. I hope so.

Way back in high school, my then-boyfriend (now husband) had set a goal to retire at age fifty. I thought he was crazy – what seventeen-year-old thinks about retirement? But he was serious, and I'm glad I stuck with him. He actually retired *before* age fifty!

When my fiftieth birthday came around, I retired, too -- well, sort of. It was at this time that I started my own part-time business as an Independent Diabetes Consultant. No, we're not millionaires, but we're comfortable. We're happy, and we're where we want to be. And that's a pretty good definition of success.

Enemy, Neighbor, Dancer, Teacher

When I was first diagnosed with diabetes, once I got past the "Why me?" stage, my relationship with diabetes was pretty clear: diabetes was the enemy and we were at war. (It was a quiet war because "being perfect" is a quiet way of life.) The object was to beat the enemy, to win. I would know I was winning because I would not get all those awful things that happened to my grandma. Of course, it would take years to know if the awful things would happen, but I was unshakable in my belief: I would be perfect, I *could* do it, and I *would* win.

I don't remember exactly when my relationship with diabetes evolved to a new stage. I think I was in my twenties; it might have been before the *grand mal* seizure, or maybe just after. I no longer thought of diabetes as the enemy, but I couldn't say diabetes was my friend, exactly; it was more like an annoying neighbor. I did my thing (as perfectly as possible), and diabetes did its thing, and we mostly stayed out of each other's way most of the time. We were civil to each other, but not friendly. It wasn't great, but it was more comfortable than being enemies. The relationship was less harsh.

After a while, my relationship with diabetes got a little closer. I remember reading an article in a diabetes newsletter long ago about how someone thought of diabetes as their dancing partner. It came to me that this was really true – diabetes wasn't living in a bunker on the other side of a hill far away, and it wasn't a neighbor living down the street. Diabetes was right there: in your space, holding your hands, moving with you all the time. It's like Fred Astaire and Ginger Rogers in the old black and white movies, which is why I started calling my diabetes "Fred."

Sometimes, despite my attempts to do everything perfectly, *Fred* stepped on my toes. Sometimes, I stepped on his.

It made me smile to think about life as a dance, with me and *Fred* dancing through it together. By this time, I had come to realize that everything about diabetes affects my life, and everything about my life affects my diabetes. *Fred* and I were partners, a team. While I would never have chosen *Fred* as a friend, somehow we had been chosen to dance together. Despite it all, we were doing a good job together, and it was comfortable.

I keep getting older (maybe wiser), and this relationship keeps shifting. *Fred* has changed over time in a subtle way from "dancing partner" to teacher.

After thirty years of living with diabetes, I hosted a "Diabetes Celebration" for our community. I had no complications – zero, nada, zilch -- from diabetes, whereas my grandmother, after thirty years with her diabetes, was in the last two years of her life and declining fast.

This was a moment I had waited a long time for, and of course I wanted to celebrate my success -- my triumph, if you will. But I also wanted to show the community that it was possible; that they, too, could choose to be lucky and successful with diabetes. And I wanted them to know that diabetes is not a monster, but a *teacher*.

To do that, we created a Community Diabetes Quilt. Each attendee at the big Celebration was given a fabric square and a felt marker and asked to answer the question, "What has diabetes taught you?"

The answers on that quilt were just amazing, and they revealed the breadth of relationships that people have with diabetes. These answers express many sentiments. Here are just a few:

"If it tastes good, spit it out!"

"You will lose your feet."

"To appreciate my wellness and empathize with others," and

"We are all in control of our destiny," while my own square in the Community Diabetes Quilt read, "To let go of perfection."

It seems funny, but through all the changes in my relationship with diabetes, I never stopped doing my diabetes self-care as perfectly as I could. But my understanding of what self-care means has changed as I became better educated and as the science of diabetes has changed over time. I realized that it wasn't the things I do that changed, but *my whole attitude and approach to living*.

Through my work helping other people with diabetes, I learned that the goal is *improvement*, not perfection. For most people, if perfection is your goal, that means you're living most of your life feeling like a failure. Or you're like me, doing the "perfect" things, then feeling betrayed because you still don't get "perfect" results.

It has been thirty-six years now since I was first diagnosed, and as odd as this may sound, I am grateful for having diabetes. Through my experiences with diabetes, I truly learned how to live a healthy life, and how to appreciate all the wonders of the human body when it works properly on its own. I have also learned to appreciate all that I have, even when it falls short of being "perfect." In many ways, I have grown to understand that we are all perfect just as we are.

If we fall short of health, and the behaviors that keep us as healthy as we can be, we are still okay.

To be human and to be alive is a gift, a joy, and a delight. When you truly see the wonders of the body, when you're grateful for how fragile and wonderful it is, it becomes easier to do all the right things to stay healthy. There doesn't need to be any effort or sense of discipline at all, providing that those things are done with respect and gratitude, and with a sense of caring for this wonderful gift (your own human body).

Because of diabetes, I have learned to love and appreciate life, to care for my body and let go of perfection, and I have learned how to help other people to improve their lives.

I still don't say that diabetes is my friend, exactly; it goes deeper than that. Diabetes is my *teacher* – a particularly hard teacher. It will keep giving me lessons until I master them, and then it will keep giving the same lessons to see if I can learn even more. More importantly, diabetes is a part of *me*. It's part of my river of life, right along with my parents and grandparents, as it helped to shape me every bit as much as they did.

I could not be the person I am without diabetes. Thanks in large part to my diabetes, I am a successful woman.

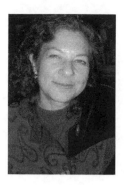

Chapter 6 *by Riva Greenberg*

You Can Go Anywhere from Here

My current work in diabetes wouldn't give you a clue about my early social awkwardness, but I was a very shy kid growing up. When I travel around the world, people often say to me, "You don't sound like you're from New York." My reply is, "That's because I never spoke as a child." The reason this is relevant is because today, I spend a great deal of my time standing in front of big groups of people, talking about diabetes awareness and other health concerns.

How I manage my diabetes today doesn't reveal my far-from-stellar beginning. Let's just say that the doctor who attended me in the hospital upon my diagnosis of type 1 diabetes in 1972 was vociferous in his insistence that I would encounter every major diabetes complication sooner or later, so I may as well know right now what I *was going* to get. I spent my second day in the hospital staring at the grey walls. I desperately tried, with little success, to stop the "Why me?" tape that kept looping in my head.

Then my doctor put two books in my hands. Each book assured me that I would go blind, lose a limb, get a heart attack, go on kidney dialysis and never have children. You might imagine after having this experience that I left the hospital depressed, but I didn't. Rather, I ended up heading for two places at the same time: one geographic, the other emotional.

The geographic place is the easier one to describe, as I went back to school, 419 miles away from my family. I was a college freshman; I arrived back on campus with vials of insulin, syringes, alcohol swabs and urine test strips. As if all of that stuff wasn't bad enough to deal with, a half-sized refrigerator, used to keep my insulin cold, moved into my dorm room like a third roommate.

As I pulled the blanket up over my legs at night to sleep, I was haunted by the notion that I would go blind. This would be frightening for anyone. I knew in my case that it really bothered me, as I was only eighteen years old and planned to be an art teacher. Worse yet, I spent several years after my diagnosis feeling a tingling, somewhat burning sensation in my right calf, which only added to my fears that something was badly wrong.

The other place I went, the emotional one, was into denial. After all, what teenager wants to believe, or even *can* believe, that her young life is ending? Especially as only a few months before, her life had shown such great promise?

Being able now to look over four decades with diabetes, I can say with relief and equanimity that I have experienced only a few minor complications: two "frozen shoulders," a slow growing cataract (after seven years my ophthalmologist tells me it's still growing so slowly there's nothing to do), minor neuropathy in one calf that disappeared and some hearing loss. Yet, I have not had any major complications – nor do I expect or intend to. My younger self, so frightened for my future, has learned that I have the capacity to create my best health.

The bad news was that when I was diagnosed, I had an awful doctor – one with no bedside manner and few facts – and he ended up scaring me so much that I didn't pay as much attention to my diabetes the first decade I had it as I should have. Of course, back in those days, ignoring my diabetes was easy to do as home glucose meters hadn't yet come onto the market. We patients had little information available to us and we didn't even know that all carbohydrates raise blood sugar not just apple pie, candy bars, and table sugar. I was advised to take insulin once a day.

The good news is that as more information came out about diabetes, I learned more about how to change my eating habits and improve my diabetes management skills. I would even bring things I'd read about to my doctor.

Looking back, I regard my transformation as somewhat remarkable, yet not uncommon: I went from being a patient who knew so little and had been made to fear so much to someone who knew a great deal, including the fact that fear alone will never help you.

When I left the hospital after being diagnosed with diabetes, I had the feeling that I no longer knew what my life was. My life felt foreign, alien to me – worst of all, like someone else's life. After all, with diabetes, there were needles and a new eating regimen involved, things I'd never before had to deal with. I remember wondering how long I'd live, since I'd heard that people with diabetes had shorter lifespans.

There was no such thing as a blood glucose meter during my first dozen years with diabetes. Twice a year, I'd go to a lab and have my blood sugar tested. This was a worthless exercise, for sure.

When I first got a meter, not only did it resemble a brick and take two minutes to read my blood sugar, it showed my blood sugar was usually around 200 mg/dL. So I know I couldn't have been very well-controlled during my first decade with diabetes.

I'd grown up a first-born child with every one of the hallmark characteristics. I was a model child: responsible, uncomplaining and hard working, so perhaps it's not surprising that I rarely told anyone I had diabetes. I didn't want to burden anyone, including my family, and I didn't think anyone could understand what it felt like to live with my fear and worry. As I learned more and started to take better care of myself, the fear and worry subsided; however, I still didn't talk about it. I kept thinking, *Who else, besides me, can understand the constant micro-management type 1 diabetes demands?*

At age twenty-eight, after working in New York City as an advertising copywriter for four years and participating in a training series having to do with personal growth, I left my job to create my own inspirational greeting cards. I wanted to inspire people to believe in themselves and their gifts. I worked out of my apartment, sitting at a little drawing board in the corner of my tiny living room. I both designed and wrote the cards. Then I'd walk around Manhattan, stick my head into a greeting card store and force myself to talk with the owner.

I loved the work. I felt inspiring people to love themselves and go after their dream was why I was put here. And for a time, I saw some success: at one point, there were around eighty-six stores that were selling my cards nationally. Almost all of the stores were based in Manhattan and Long Island, where my father was selling them out of the trunk of his car, while one store sold them in Seattle (that store run by two lovely sisters I had met on a trip there). But after four years, this starving artist needed a full-time job to pay the rent.

Leafing through a trade magazine, I saw an ad for English-language copywriters wanted for a Japanese advertising agency in Tokyo. I thought that would be a great adventure and applied. Eight months later I was headed to Tokyo. I packed up my belongings and moved to a place I'd never been, where I didn't speak the language, couldn't read anything and didn't think about what it would mean to be a Western woman in a traditional Japanese company, let alone a woman with diabetes.

Looking back on this time in my life, I realize that although I was told diabetes would be my downfall, I never let it stop me from doing anything. I never believed it would (or should), and it never has.

63

I actually became known as my Japanese company's "secret weapon." Honestly! There's an old, discolored issue of *U.S. News & World Report* somewhere that I'm sure I could dig up that says so. I was such a novelty in 1986 – an American woman working for a traditional Japanese advertising agency – that I was news! I lived in Tokyo for six years, traveled extensively, and the hardest thing I remember about having diabetes was managing to avoid the staples of an Asian diet – mounds of rice and noodles!

Living in Japan changed many things for me. The first was that I stopped doing one of the earliest things I had been taught to do for my diabetes. The first day at work, I went to the company clinic for alcohol swabs. Lo and behold, they had no such thing. Instead, a confused looking Japanese woman handed me a giant-sized bottle of alcohol and a bag of puffy, white cotton balls. The balls left rivers of alcohol running down my leg, so I stopped using them. I haven't used an alcohol swab since; I read some years ago that you shouldn't because they dry out the skin.

The other change Japan brought was that, on my own time, I began to write and illustrate a book I titled, *The ABCs of Loving Yourself.* I returned to my greeting card roots to draw whimsical characters and write one-liners of inspirational text for each letter of the alphabet. I sold the book to Random House in Sydney, Australia, where it was published. However, my editor told me he thought the drawings were "too sweet" for the Australian market, so he bought the text only; I was left with a full collection of unpublished A to Z illustrations. The book won the Australian Children's Book Award the year it was printed, but the leftover images that the editor hadn't wanted would become worth even more to me down the road.

Returning home to New York, now thirty-eight years old, I found a good doctor and began to pay more attention to my diabetes care. I made two critical changes at the time. I began practicing the "Don't finish what's on your plate" eating plan. I'd leave over something each time I had a plate of food in front of me. It could be one spoonful, but I determined this is how I would begin to eat less and lose some weight. I also began walking to and from work, forty-five minutes each way. Subsequently, my diabetes, and life, improved.

Another event that year also helped me embrace both my diabetes and myself. I flew to London, where the Australian man I was then dating lived. He knew I had diabetes and I thought he understood what was involved. But I was wrong entirely, or at least wrong about what he was willing to take on.

One night I awoke in his flat with low blood sugar. In the dark, I maneuvered myself over his body toward the kitchen in order to find something sweet. "What's happening?" he asked sleepily.

"I need sugar," I replied. He didn't really seem to get what was wrong, and instead rolled back to sleep. I found two shortbread cookies in his kitchen without ever turning on the light, but as I munched in the darkness a different light turned on: the one in my head. I realized that if someone who professed to love me could leave me feeling so unsafe, then I needed to be on my own side and take good care of myself.

This "a-ha moment" led me to tell all my friends about my diabetes. They were curious, sympathetic, supportive, and conveyed their feelings with words like these, "I love you. Please let me know if you need anything. It's no big deal."

I still wasn't convinced, however, that a man would ever love me enough to marry me and take on my diabetes with its possible complications and an uncertain future. Of course, I was wrong about that. Meeting the right man is actually what launched the work I do today.

At forty-eight years old, four events happened that changed the course of this second chapter of my life, and turned out to be blessings in disguise.

First, I lost my job, as I'd been working for a Website development company that went bankrupt.

Second, I went into the hospital for "frozen shoulder" surgery. (My shoulder is perfect now, by the way.)

Third, I got married, *not* to the Australian, but to a Dutchman. Now, if I stir in the night, my husband will immediately ask, "Are you okay? Can I get you juice or your meter?" (He also carries SweeTarts ™ and glucose tablets in his pockets in case I go low.) My husband has become a staunch supporter of my work.

The last of the four significant events that occurred that year was that I went to see a diabetes educator for the first time in thirty-two years. I did so because now, my health was important to someone else besides me.

After my first visit with the educator, I thought about becoming a diabetes educator myself. But learning that I would first need to have an advanced degree in medicine, psychology, pharmacology, physical therapy or exercise, then practice for 1,000 hours before I could become certified was daunting.

As I felt that was not my road, I began to look for a copywriter job again. It was what I knew. Trouble was, I also knew I didn't want to do it anymore. I wanted to do what I'd *always* hoped to do – help other people believe in themselves and create more fulfilling lives.

It was my incredibly loving, bright, and supportive husband who said to me, "You're a writer. You'd like to help others who have diabetes. So why don't you write about what it's like to live with diabetes?"

I looked at him sweetly, rolled my eyes, and said, "Honey, who's going to buy a book about what *I think* about living with diabetes?" So instead, I began to interview other people with diabetes, their loved ones, and diabetes professionals, because I thought that would make a pretty good book –

65

a collection of stories. It hasn't become a book – yet – but I have interviewed more than 150 people to date and continue to work on it.

In the meantime, I've had two other diabetes books published: *50 Diabetes Myths That Can Ruin Your Life and the 50 Diabetes Truths That Can Save It*, and *The ABC's Of Loving Yourself With Diabetes*.

My road to where I am today began in the spring of 2004 with a road map. My husband and I sat on a park bench one afternoon and wrote down my vision, which was to help educate and inspire others with diabetes to better manage their condition and live happier lives. That vision sat in the center of a large, blank white sheet of paper. Then we drew colored lines coming out, going in all directions to various steps and paths to pursue that would lead to my dream.

Step number one was to write a column for a diabetes magazine. One day after reviewing the four major diabetes magazines, I called the editor of *Diabetes Health* and told her I wanted to write a column. I talked for about twenty minutes about my background and what that column might be like. She said she would call me back in two hours after she reviewed my Website and some articles I'd directed her to that I'd written. When she actually called me back in two hours with the go-ahead, I was shocked and nervous. I ended up writing for *Diabetes Health* for two years. Now, I write a regular column on diabetes and health for the *Huffington Post.*

Step number two was to write and illustrate a book that would help people with the emotional side of diabetes, which I did in 2007. As you may have figured out from my previous reference, this book is called *The ABCs of Loving Yourself with Diabetes*. It took me six months to write. (I was so excited by the idea of this book that I spent much of my vacation in Holland, after I had started the book, scribbling pages rather than focused on the bicyclists and canals. I still remember scribbling one page while eating an omelet in a café in Brussels, as I watched the rain come down in sheets against the windows.)

My husband is a computer geek. Shortly after we got married, he urged me to scan all my artwork into my computer. There they were, the drawings I had done seventeen years ago for my first book, *The ABCs of Loving Yourself,* looking up at me and saying, "We knew you wouldn't abandon us!" Those are the pictures now in *The ABCs of Loving Yourself with Diabetes*.

I wasn't able to interest a publisher in picking up *The ABCs of Loving Yourself with Diabetes* because it is not a traditional book about diabetes, but I felt so strongly about it that I chose to publish it myself. I think of this book as my manifesto; it coaches readers to develop the emotional resilience to "keep on keepin' on" with their diabetes care by helping to energize more of their positive emotions.

In 2009, I manned a table all the way in the back of the huge Exhibition Hall at the International Diabetes Federation World Congress in Montreal. I had pre-arranged to give away 1,000 copies each of *The ABCs of Loving Yourself with Diabetes* and *50 Diabetes Myths That Can Ruin Your Life and the 50 Diabetes Truths That Can Save It*. It was my gift to the health care providers who attended the conference, a way of saying "thank you" to those who help us take care of ourselves. It was a delight to give away and sign the books, while watching the convention-goers' appreciation due to receiving such an unexpected gift. I expected the books to last until the fourth day of the conference, but they were gone by 11:00 AM on the second day!

In one of my greeting cards back in 1980 I wrote, "The world is nothing more than what you make it . . . and nothing less." I still believe that. The quality of our lives is often determined by what we do and how we live in the world. While we all face challenges, how we respond to them is what's important. Like the joy I received from the convention-goers, and the joy those who unexpectedly took home my books experienced, we can change our own and others' lives by stepping out and sharing our gifts.

Step number three was to give talks to other patients with diabetes and medical staff. I do that now across the country by speaking at conferences and facilitating workshops as a patient-expert and researcher in our capacity to flourish with diabetes, and create lives of greater health and happiness. For example, last year I spoke to forty health care providers at one hospital in Singapore, and two hundred health care providers at another hospital in Singapore.

I'm also a peer-mentor, and I travel across the country speaking to groups of patients at support groups and health fairs about managing their diabetes. The most powerful part of this program is that people are hearing about diabetes from *me*, another patient. I knew I wanted to participate in this program as soon as I heard about it, but when I called I was told they weren't taking any new candidates. Six calls, one every month, put me in the next training session six months later. While there's still that shy girl inside of me (my husband has to push me out the door to go to a party where I don't know anyone), a certain determination has always been inside of me, too, when I truly believe in something or the rightness of something.

My desire to work in this field was always to help people manage the emotional side of diabetes, to build the inner strength and stamina to get up every day and do those things we need to do to take care of ourselves for the long haul. While our health care providers are trained to cut and cure, they receive very little, if any, training to guide, coach and support people to live a full and flourishing life with a chronic illness.

67

Many health care providers also, because they don't know any better, try scaring patients into taking care of their diabetes. They think this works, but it doesn't. We can't look very long at what we hope to avoid, so fear works only temporarily (if at all).

What does work, however, is to learn all you can, look toward where you *want* to go – have an idealized vision of yourself and your future – and head there. You need to notice and appreciate what you're doing well, take baby steps to improve those things you aren't doing so well, and dig deep for answers as to why it's worth it to you to do the work of taking care of yourself. Then keep those answers close at hand and refer to them as needed.

Contrary to popular belief, our history does not have to be our future – not when we decide it will not be. And we can remake ourselves when we commit to walking a different path. Consider that at eighteen, I was told my life would be dismal by now. I now use that false information to tell audiences, "You can have a great life, not *despite* diabetes, but *because* of it – if you use diabetes to get healthier, appreciate what you *do* have and find your meaning and purpose in life."

I am certain the decisions I began making twenty years ago to take care of my diabetes – eating healthy food, eating smaller portions and walking an hour a day have made me healthier than I would be had I never gotten diabetes. Checking and correcting my blood sugar more often has helped to keep my blood sugar within the target range, and rounding up a posse of friends with diabetes has made me insanely happier.

I began this work eight years ago. These days, I say with a chuckle, "I'm in the eighth year of my twenty year overnight success." Yet when I look back, I see all the threads that have led me here and have prepared me to do what I'm doing today: I grew up an observer and listener; I developed my talent for writing and drawing; I became interested in studying self-growth, psychology and spirituality; I always questioned myself as to why I was here and what I was meant to do; I've consistently learned about how to improve my diabetes management; I kept those little drawings that never got thrown away. And last but not least, I reached fifty years of age, where you care less about what other people think, and feel freer to say exactly what *you* think.

Today, my work is about something significant I noticed when I was interviewing others with diabetes: people tend to live from one of two mindsets. In other words, people either mostly "cope" with diabetes, or they "flourish" with diabetes. Or to put it another way, people either saw themselves as victims and were struggling with a sense of loss and feeling overwhelmed, or they had created a life where diabetes was just a part of it.

These latter people used diabetes as a spur, something which would force them to re-examine what was important to them and begin to follow their dreams. Many in the second category lost weight they couldn't lose before and got more active, while for some, walking around the block morphed into running marathons. Some experienced greater self-worth by teaching and supporting family members where diabetes is rampant. Most became more caring and compassionate, because they know that many others deal with something worse. Almost all of the second group felt diabetes either hadn't impacted their happiness or had actually increased it.

In 2008, I entered the "Inspired by Diabetes" competition sponsored by Eli Lilly and the International Diabetes Federation. The competition asked you to express how diabetes had an impact on your life. I created a poster of myself using a picture a friend had taken where I happen to be standing with my shoulders back and arms folded as if in a stance of triumph and I wrote an essay titled, "The Antidote to Diabetes – Living Proud." I won First Prize.

How we hold our diabetes determines, to a great extent, how we experience it. If you can feel proud of how you manage and live with diabetes, you will feel more positive and give diabetes less weight. Recently I heard Jay Hewitt, an ironman tri-athlete with type 1 diabetes, say this: "Make the bad thing that happened to you the best thing that's happened to you." I couldn't agree more.

I am a "recovering perfectionist," so it's not always easy living with a condition I cannot control. And for everyone who shouts, "I control my diabetes, it doesn't control me!" I disagree (there's that cantankerous fifty-eight-year-old!). We *cannot* control diabetes. As I'm sure you've learned, it has a mind of its own. But we can do our best to *manage* it by deciding how we live with it, and with that, we can have our best health and *most* of our sanity.

I take four to six injections a day and do seven to ten blood sugar tests a day. I have some minor complications and there's always the chance I may get more. At times, living with diabetes is frustrating, wearying, sad, and it continues to test me, but at the same time, it has bestowed blessings – for example, I am certain that I enjoy better health than I would if I'd never gotten diabetes. I appreciate all that I have: my family and friends, my work, being fit, a good movie or book, a great glass of wine, a day in the country without mosquitoes, the support and pride I see reflected back to me in my husband's eyes and the joy of helping others.

When my husband and I got engaged ten years ago, I told him in a moment of benceficence, "You can back out now if you want to. My diabetes will make our life more uncertain. I don't know what my future will be and I never want to burden you with that."

He wrapped his loving arms around me and said, "You're with me now, and I'm with you." And that's how it's been.

From that moment I made an unshakeable decision: I want to live the healthiest life I can for as long as I can, and I will do whatever it takes to have it.

Today, I am the author of three books. I write articles that I hope make people think. I speak across the country, and I travel – and play – across the world. Diabetes and I have been across North America, through much of Europe, Asia, Australia, New Zealand, even Iceland and the Soviet Union! And I'm *still* not sure how to adjust my insulin for crossing times zones other than constant testing the first few days.

I'm always developing new materials and I have a philosophy, a curriculum, and a coaching system for designing a healthy, happy life with diabetes – a life where we can use our diabetes as a stimulus to live bigger, yet treasure everything small. Oh, yes – I use the moments someone sees me injecting insulin, or when a stewardess serves me a "diabetic breakfast" of pancakes, syrup, fruit yogurt and orange juice as "teachable moments." (Not to mention an opportunity to get 15,000 free frequent flier miles for such a *big* mistake!)

I am called an inspirational speaker because I encourage others with diabetes to look up and see their possibilities. It's not so different than when I was drawing my cards in 1980 in a little corner of my little apartment, except everything I wanted to use inside of me, and do, is now on a bigger stage. I believe with all my heart, my soul, and sometimes a few sore fingers that you can have a great life not *despite* diabetes but *because* of it. I know I have.

I am hopeful about all the improvements that are coming down the pike to make life with diabetes better and easier. When people say, "Don't get your hopes up," I reply, "Get them up and keep them up!" because hope is a powerful force.

An acquaintance recently said to me, "You live with your illness with such grace." I was dumbstruck, because I think people are hardly ever aware of my diabetes. Sometimes I feel frustrated that people don't see all that I do to manage my diabetes so I can stay as well as possible for as long as possible. But maybe that is how a chronic disease should look: it is just a part of you, sometimes the worst, but also sometimes the best.

I often have said since I took up this work, "The Universe keeps dropping gifts at my feet." My husband replies, "Don't discount all the hard work you've done." I don't, yet I'm convinced that being on the right track, leading with your heart, and following with your feet – whatever that is for you – opens more doors than you can possibly imagine.

The ultimate reward, for me, can be summed up by something Mahatma Gandhi said, "Happiness is when what you think, what you say, and what you do are in harmony." I am happy, because my work is an extension of my life:

I write, speak, and teach from my everyday experiences. I have a partner who loves and supports me. And there's little that makes me happier than helping others.

While I don't generally make New Year's resolutions, last year I resolved to "Be Bold." I decided to go after what I wanted, and by doing so, it unearthed opportunities I would not otherwise have had. That's why this year, I've resolved to "Be Bolder!"

I never did have that baby I was told I couldn't have, but not because I couldn't. Rather, somehow I sensed that I was here to influence the many rather than the few. In that spirit, I hope my story will help you realize that, like so many others, you *can* live well with diabetes.

So this is my story since that fateful day when I heard I had a debilitating disease that I would live with for the rest of my life.

As you look forward, also look back to what you've accomplished over the years. It will help you see your strengths and capabilities to move forward with diabetes. As you do, you, too, may find that there's a blessing in your diabetes, and see that you can *use* it to make your life brighter, bigger, and better that you ever dreamed.

Website: www.DiabetesStories.com
Website: www.DiabetesbyDesign.com

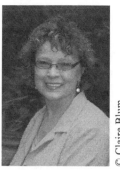

© Claire Blum

Chapter 7　　*by Connie Hanham-Cain, RN, CDE*

Diabetes Consciousness: A Journey of Mind-Body Self-Awareness

Diagnosis: Diabetes

I have lived in a body with type 1 diabetes since the winter of 1962-1963, as I was diagnosed when I was eight years old. In the early days of my diagnosis, the disease was called "sugar diabetes" or "juvenile diabetes" and "brittle diabetes." I never liked those terms, because use of the term "juvenile" made me think of juvenile delinquents. Worse yet, whenever I heard grown-ups using the term "brittle diabetic," it was used to indicate "bad diabetes." Both terms conjured up an image of me being labeled as a "bad diabetic." I knew that I had diabetes, so why did it need to be labeled as either juvenile or brittle?

I was diagnosed in the third grade. My parents had divorced the year before, after which my younger brother, Billy, and I lived with our mother, Lillian, in a two-bedroom duplex apartment on a busy city street in the stately Old West End neighborhood in Toledo, Ohio. Mom worked five to six days a week as a dance teacher/choreographer. My dad, who was unemployed due to unresolved alcoholism, had Saturday visitation rights with us.

My divorced, resourceful single mom pretty much raised us by herself with the help of high school and college-age dance students as babysitters. She also employed a housekeeper two days a week. Sometimes my maternal grandmother would come from Chicago to live with us for a few weeks at a time to visit and help my mom out.

73

Prior to my young life being altered with the diagnosis of type 1 diabetes, I spent my early childhood going to school. I read children's books, rode my bike, played with neighborhood kids, took dance classes and rehearsed for dance theatre performance productions, and of course spent time with my family during the holidays. Billy and I were educated in Roman Catholic schools, but because my mother's family practiced the Eastern Orthodox Byzantine Rite, we celebrated both the Roman and the Eastern Orthodox holidays.

In 1962, mom was hired as a Cultural Arts Specialist at the Toledo Jewish Community Center. At this point, we started to celebrate all the Jewish holidays, by proxy, as well. The common thread I realized at a very early age is that all three spiritual traditions recognized the same angels and prayed to the same God.

My spiritual journey with diabetes started in church. It happened while I was attending daily mass with my third grade class. It was time to go up to the altar to receive communion, and I felt too sick to go. My head was pounding with a splitting headache, my body felt heavy and I was nauseated. I was sweating profusely and felt like I was burning up.

As the other little girls moved out of the church pew to go to communion, I slid down to the center of the pew and I proceeded to vomit, urinate, and lose my bowels all at the same time. I remember trembling and shivering as I buried my face in my hands, crying and praying to God to forgive me for making a mess in church. I prayed that He please heal me, let me go home and keep me safe. Sister St. Therese, my third grade teacher, came and gently carried me out of the pew. The next thing I remember is my mom as she took me home.

The next few days or weeks are a blur. I remember being kept out of school; my homework assignments were brought to me each day by a sixth grade neighbor. I know that I went to see several doctors to determine what was wrong. In the meantime, my grandmother arrived from Chicago to spend Christmas with us.

One day during this interlude, I was doing math homework and was having difficulty understanding a multiplication problem. I went to ask my mom for help. She was sitting at the kitchen table with her back to the door that separated the bedroom from the kitchen. My grandmother stood over her, comforting her. My mom was crying and hitting her hand against the table while she sobbed, "They don't know what's wrong with her. She might have anemia, or leukemia, or she might have diabetes."

Mom and Grandma did not see me in the doorway, so I slowly and quietly backed away to return to my desk in the living room. I folded my hands on the desk and sat there for a moment while I thought about what I had just heard. I knew that children died from leukemia and people with anemia had something wrong with their blood that made them faint. But I had never heard of diabetes.

I then talked to God again. I prayed, "Please, God, if I have to be sick, whatever is wrong with me, give me something I can live with so I don't die as a child. Please don't make my mom sad and break her heart. Give me a good life. I promise I'll be good."

Shortly after Christmas that year, I went into Riverside Hospital for a three-week inpatient stay. This was necessary because both mom and I needed to learn about the lifetime, and life-sustaining, practice of giving insulin injections. We were also told about the "diabetic diet" exchange list as we adjusted to my life with diabetes.

Awareness of Choice with Diabetes

As a young child and adolescent growing up with diabetes, I faced the usual lifestyle challenges that every kid with diabetes must face. For my mother and me, it meant getting up extra early every morning before school to test my urine, boil the syringes, and to eat a carefully prepared and measured breakfast. I never had the appetite to eat all the food that I was required to eat, but my mom wouldn't let me leave the table until I ate everything that was prepared and placed on my "diabetic diet" plate. It sometimes took me well over an hour to eat everything and I came to despise the words "you *have* to eat because you're a diabetic." Eating and "diabetic" meal portions became a power struggle between my mom and me, and for the most part, as a kid, I did not enjoy measured meal times. However, for the first few years of living with diabetes, I stuck to the "no candies and cookies" rule and did not "cheat eat." (That word concept still annoys me!)

One day, at age ten or eleven, I was home from school alone for the day after a wicked insulin reaction in the early morning hours of the night before. My mom kept me home from school to let me sleep off the aftermath of a severe *hypoglycemic* seizure. I awoke from a nap and felt hungry, so I went to the refrigerator to see what was there to eat. I noticed a tin of English tea cookies that mom had received as a gift from one of her students. Curious, I looked inside and what I saw was very appealing: chocolate and vanilla sandwich cookies with a vanilla cream filling. They looked and smelled so good, much better than the sugar-free gelatin or weird tasting sugar-free candies or bland sugar-free cookies that I was usually given as a snack. I wasn't in the mood for graham crackers and milk this time; I wanted a real cookie!

I remember that I struggled internally whether or not to "sneak" a cookie. In my mind, I heard my mom and my relatives saying "You can't eat sugar anymore or you could die!" I looked at the cookies and savored the vanilla smell of them for quite awhile before I reached in and took one. I hid it under my pajama top, scurried back to the bedroom, and dove under the covers holding my precious, forbidden treat. I smelled it, licked it, and slowly began to nibble on it, savoring the lusciousness of the rich vanilla taste and the smooth creaminess of the frosting layer.

All the while, an inner dialogue was going on between my "good" versus "bad" diabetes self. I thought, *If I am going to die from eating this cookie, then I want to really enjoy and savor the experience.* I felt pleasure as I tasted every nibble, but afterward I waited to die. I felt ashamed and guilty over breaking the taboo of "no sweets." I waited for God to take me because I had "cheated". But what promise had I broken? Had I taken a vow to be a "good diabetic"?

After lying under the covers awhile longer, I realized that I felt fine. I didn't die, nor was I going to die from eating that cookie. So I got up, went to the refrigerator and got another one, and scurried back into the bedroom to hide under the covers to eat the second one. I satisfied my "cookie urge" and I was still alive.

This episode activated a lifelong inner dialogue, that's still ongoing, of consciously being aware of choosing what, or what not, to eat. Somehow, in my eleven-year-old mind, I came to understand that I had a choice in what I eat, be it "good' or "bad." For the first time, I realized that I could either make good choices, or I could make less than good choices. The choice was up to me and my diabetes consciousness.

I Exist, Therefore I Am

What is diabetes consciousness? For me, an early, profound, and life-changing experience of living with diabetes is what has taught me about the mind-body connection as a vehicle for consciousness.

When I was a child (and again as an adolescent), I suffered through several episodes of severe *hypoglycemia*, resulting in seizures. During an episode, my body sat in a chair, convulsing. My brother, Billy, would try to hold me still at the shoulders while my mom poured orange juice and Karo syrup down my throat to get glucose into my body. (This took place in the days before home *glucagon* kits were readily available.)

I was completely aware of myself as "a thinking and feeling entity," but I was disconnected from being inside my body. My consciousness, my true "I Am" self, or what you might think of as the divine life presence that lives inside my body, was fully intact during those times. I expanded as large as the area of the kitchen walls, so large as to be hitting myself on the boundaries of the kitchen ceiling. I experienced floating and reaching through space and an odd, curious timelessness as I aimed my conscious mind to anchor itself back into the contours and confines of my physical body. I experienced the "All That I Am" consciousness as being tethered to my physical presence by a luminous cord of a pulsating and shimmering substance. It had an elasticity that functioned like a bungee cord; it would snap up and down in every direction.

I willed my consciousness to get back into my body. I remember trying to step up into a moving train in the space/time continuum of a starry universe – this is as close as I can come to explaining this experience. As I neared the moving train to step on to it, my consciousness passed right through it – right through my body! I continued to rise and fall through the starry field. I heard tonal sounds that sounded like harmonious chords of "Ommmmm." I felt completely connected to *my truest self.*

As my blood sugar stabilized, I experienced my *self* re-entering my body through the top of my head and into my solar plexus. I could then see through the eyes in my head, hear sounds around me through my ears and feel the sensation of being fully anchored into my physical body once again.

My mom would peel off my wet clothes and throw me into a warm bubble bath. She washed away all the sticky juice and syrup she'd used to bring me back. The hot soak in the tub helped to calm my cold and clammy *post-hypoglycemic* shivers until I was warm enough to dry off, put on clean pajamas, and go back to bed.

Those exhausting episodes taught me that *I exist* and *I am alive*, wholly within my body and outside of my body. Later in my life, these out-of-body experiences led me to realize that "I Am" is a state of Being that exists eternally and has nothing to do with whether I have diabetes or not.

Diabetes has blessed me by enabling me to see and experience that "I Am" state, which is both terrifying and blissful at the same time. The terrifying part is the sense of losing control as my blood sugar drops and I have to struggle to stay conscious in order to take care of myself. I have a perception of knowing that there is a fine thread that could snap instantly if my blood glucose drops too low; that means my experience of living in this lifetime could be over in that same instant. (I have been very fortunate: I am still here.) The blissful part is the profound sense of *Eternal inner calm, oneness and peace* that diabetes has privileged me to see, in glimpses, through the perceptions of fluctuating blood glucose levels.

Experiences of Awakening, Near-Death, and Rebirth

As a kid, I learned wholesome and healthy self-care skills while attending Camp Zanika diabetes sleep-away camp in Ohio for two weeks every June during my childhood and adolescence. Camp Zanika shaped the course of life with diabetes very early in my journey because we kids had a unique "special something" that bonded us all together.

Through camp, my diabetes consciousness was activated and reinforced. I became more aware of *hypoglycemia* and knew that it was better to choose healthy-looking food that was green, colorful and tasted fresh. I blessed the food I ate before taking it into my body, and prayed that it be metabolized to the highest good to keep me healthy.

Along with that, I learned to be physically active and have fun doing "kid things" with other kids. For the first time since being diagnosed with diabetes, I experienced how to be a normal kid who happened to live in a body with diabetes.

During the 1970s and 1980s, I experienced the dawning of the "New Age" of creative thinking and spirituality, and of diabetes self-care knowledge. In my late teens and early twenties, I attended New York University (NYU) School of the Arts for three years. I studied acting, singing, and dance because I wished to have a career as a Broadway performer. Along the way, I auditioned for many shows, and was rejected by many shows.

Disappointed and disillusioned, I dropped out of NYU and got "spiritual." I started looking for answers for life's deepest questions, and I became acquainted with the esoteric spiritual traditions and meditation practices brought from the East by Russian-Greek-Armenian mystic, G.I. Gurdjieff, and British research author, J.G. Bennett, who was a long-time adherent of Gurdjieff's teachings. This "new thought psychology" originated in ancient spiritual traditions of the Near, Middle and Far East and appealed to my love of, and interest in, the sacred music and dance ceremonies of world cultures. I began a lifelong journey on the Path of Enlightenment as a seeker and practitioner of spiritual knowledge and truth.

I don't remember much about how I managed my diabetes in those days, except for taking NPH U-80 insulin once or twice a day, as it was before the use of blood glucose meters became commonplace. At this time, I really didn't know much about the details of my diabetes except that I had it. I had the good sense to make fairly healthy choices for myself, even if I was living in the "dark ages" with regards to diabetes self-care.

Even though I pursued spiritual studies and holistic practices, I really did not have a solid clue as to what was truly going on with my diabetes. I prayed a lot, and asked God to guide me to make the right choices for my health. I read books on food combining and healing negative emotions with positive affirmations, and used color meditation and applied light therapy to energize and heal my pancreas. I juice-fasted to cleanse my body of toxins and ate a vegetarian diet. I also studied yoga and practiced sacred dance traditions.

As a young adult, I lived close to nature in a spiritual, agricultural community in West Virginia. I ate pure and healthy food; was physically active doing farm chores; and studied, taught, and performed belly dance and Eastern dance movement traditions. It was a time of deep inner searching; I practiced self-discipline with the aim of developing a higher consciousness in order to better serve as a vehicle of light in the world.

I met with many wise, spiritually mature teachers of sacred wisdom traditions. My soul was on fire to know God in the purest sense. I was inspired by the spiritual wisdom keepers I met; my heart and soul were so deeply touched with love, healing and compassion that I was changed forever. It was around this time that I started to realize my whole self, including my diabetes, is a part of my life experience: the physical, emotional, intellectual and spiritual processes that I've gone through in my life. My "diabetes self" is an integrated part of me, and an added layer of consciousness. But even realizing that, as I had due to my spiritual seeking, I knew that I still wasn't taking the best care of my diabetes.

I married a fellow seeker in 1981, and shortly thereafter became pregnant for the first time. We hadn't planned on having a child so soon in our marriage; worse yet, at that time, my diabetes was not under good control. I miscarried our baby after only six weeks.

After the devastation of losing the baby, I became depressed and despondent. Several months later, I ended up being hospitalized with *diabetic ketoacidosis* for three weeks in Long Island, NY. During that hospitalization, I was so sick and wiped out that I thought I was going to die.

One evening, I summoned enough strength to pray and ask God to please heal me. I asked to transform my ignorance of how to best live with diabetes into something positive, something I could work with. I sensed that it wasn't my time to cross over, but I knew that I had to find a way to live harmoniously with my diabetes so that I didn't cross over before my time. I prayed to live on the side of life rather than so close to the edge, near the doorway of death.

The next day during my morning shower, I felt as though I was being washed in a shower of the Holy Spirit. I heard a chorus of angels sing in perfect harmony. I wept tears of sorrow that transformed into tears of joy; I cried tears of release, rebirth, and renewal as the water poured upon me like golden, cleansing light. When I stepped out, I knew that my life was set to change.

That afternoon, a very kind and caring nurse came into my hospital room. She sat on my bed and asked me if I understood how insulin works in a body. I had to admit that after nineteen years of living with diabetes, I didn't really know. She gave me a large-print patient education manual to read called, "How Insulin Works in Type 1 Diabetes." Then she said, "I know this is written on a fourth grade reading level, but read it anyway. You never know; you may learn something useful from it." Up to that point, I had never heard of type 1 diabetes!

I read that book from cover to cover. I was both intrigued and fascinated because I felt like I was reading a manual that penetrated deep into the very life processes of the cells in my body. Because of this book, I began to realize the key tenets of diabetes self-healing. I was "born again," as both an enlightened person, and someone who'd been enlightened with regards to diabetes.

The Wonder Years and After

After the "diabetes rebirth experience" in 1982, my diabetes self-knowledge accelerated into high gear as I entered the exciting world of diabetes research and new self-care developments. We now had blood glucose meters to check our finger-stick glucose readings. Continuous infusion insulin pumps were introduced. Multiple daily insulin injections, along with the use of a blood glucose meter, were about to be phased in as the standard of treatment. The Diabetes Control and Complications Trial (DCCT) was underway and study centers were recruiting people with diabetes to participate in cutting edge research studies.

I started hanging out at the Long Island chapter of the American Diabetes Association (ADA) in order to learn as much about diabetes as I could. I attended an ADA-sponsored self-care class and a diabetes peer advocate training for volunteers to lead support groups and community outreach activities for different age groups. I was involved with young adult support groups on Long Island and in Manhattan for several years.

I met Dr. Lois Jovanovic, MD, in late 1982 through an ADA support group connection. She was conducting research studies on diabetes and pregnancy and was part of the DCCT. A "diabetes sister" who had lost a child because of complications related to her diabetes in pregnancy referred me to Dr. Lois. Because I had miscarried the year before and I was a woman with type 1 diabetes who wanted to get pregnant, I met the criteria to be selected for the study.

I met with Dr Lois and her research assistant nurse, Molly, at New York Hospital, Cornell Medical Center, for preliminary testing. Molly drew my blood and accidentally stuck herself with the needle that she had drawn my blood with. She looked at Lois; Lois looked at her. They said something about "infection control." I wasn't yet a nurse, so I did not get the full gist of what they were talking about, but I understood enough to know about the AIDS scare.

I was a bit nervous over meeting them for the first time, which might be why I chimed in, stating, "Don't worry, you can't catch anything from me – just diabetes and it's not contagious."

They both looked at one another, then at me, before laughing out loud. Dr. Lois put her arm around my shoulder and said, "The reason we are laughing with you is because we both have type 1 diabetes!"

Over the next three years, I was blessed with the privilege of being under the care of Dr. Lois in the DCCT research studies. One of my greatest gifts at that time was going through a five-day, week-long Diabetes Self-Management Education (DSME) class at the Diabetes Self-Care Center in Manhattan. I got to meet with Dr. Lois daily, and experienced personalized DSME with her incredible staff that included Barbara Turro, RD, who taught me how to count carbohydrates, two wonderful nurses, and an exercise physiologist. It was an incredible and inspiring experience that changed, and still influences, the way I manage my diabetes every day of my life.

Dr. Lois personally nurtured and mentored me for the three years that I was under her dedicated and loving care. She encouraged me to become confident in my self-care. I participated in, and learned to apply, the many tools and skills that helped me understand what to do in order to be in control of my body so I could live fully as a healthy human being who just happens to have diabetes. Unfortunately, I did not have a child under her watch, as my former husband and I divorced after three years of a very difficult marriage. (It was not meant to be.) Dr. Lois referred me to psychotherapy to deal with my depression and anxiety after the miscarriage and divorce. I spent parallel time with Dr. Viviane Lind, MD, a holistic psychiatrist based in Manhattan.

Because of the vast love and healing presence of both of these great women in my life during this emotionally difficult and enlightening time, I was inspired and influenced to become a nurse. I strive every day to teach, and provide self-healing guidance to, the patients and peers I serve with similar wisdom, understanding, and compassion that my role models Dr. Lois and Dr. Viviane shared with me.

I went back to school in 1986 to follow the calling, develop the gifts, and learn what doctors and nurses know. I wished to use what I learned in order to serve humanity as a holistic diabetes educator and mental health nurse. The next few years, I went to Rockland Community College to earn an Associate's degree in nursing. During that time, a holistic nursing instructor introduced me to Reiki, Therapeutic Touch and various concepts of energy healing. Parallel to my regular nursing school training, I apprenticed as a healer under the guidance of Rev. Ojela Frank, MSC, MSTh, and learned to apply trans-personal energy healing techniques in my work as a nurse, and on myself.

After earning my license to practice as an RN, I continued to study trans-personal psychology and energy field healing techniques with several teachers as I sought new ways to facilitate healing for other people (as well as my own diabetes). These teachers included Dora Kunz, Dr. Delores Krieger RN, PhD, Joseph Rael, and Dr. Marsha Dale Lopez, PhD.

During the 1980s, my inner spiritual life was guided and shaped by my association with Sheikh Muzaffer Ozak, aka "Efendi," and his dervishes from Istanbul and New York City. It was through my experiences as a practicing Sufi that I learned to use my diabetes as a self-regulating discipline and tool for my own spiritual transformation.

Efendi and several of the Turkish dervishes had type 2 diabetes. They asked me to teach them what I had learned about living well with diabetes during my time with Dr. Lois at the Diabetes Self-Care Program and the DCCT studies. I assisted these gentlemen in getting blood glucose meters and I taught them how to self-test and monitor their blood glucose levels. Thus, they became my first group of diabetes self-care students.

My greatest inner healing took place during the years I spent with Sheikh Muzaffer, and I wouldn't be the person that I am today without the lessons I learned from him. I was inspired by Dr. Lois and Dr. Viviane, but it was my first experiences of sharing diabetes self-care knowledge with other people who had diabetes that really motivated me to aim for a career as a Certified Diabetes Educator (CDE).

As I had a foot in both worlds, those of everyday life and of my spiritual passions, I had to find a way to manage my diabetes in both worlds. For example, during the month of Ramadan fasting, after consulting with my doctors along with Sheikh Muzaffer, I was told that, for me, ritual fasting would be unwise. An alternative approach was for me to practice being disciplined and precise in controlling my diabetes. As a spiritual practice, I was to give thanks for the gift of diabetes, even if it seemed to be a burden, because, in essence, it was a gift from God.

The Sufi belief is that everything happens for a reason, and everything comes from God: the good and the bad alike, ultimately for the highest good. After understanding this, I felt a calling to serve as a healing agent and coach, to teach and guide people on how to live consciously, healthfully, and responsibly in their bodies. It took me many years to earn my certification as a CDE, because this was a circuitous route. But somehow, I always ended up serving as a diabetes resource nurse in clinical settings.

As a nurse healer professional, I have earned many specialty certifications, but the one I am most proud of is RN, CDE, which I earned in 2006. My current job is with the Visiting Nurse Service of Schenectady and Saratoga Counties as Diabetes Resource Coordinator. I serve as a community-based diabetes educator, and I see people with diabetes in their homes or settings where they live, work, and socialize. I returned to college in 2010 and will complete my Bachelor of Science in Nursing degree through the University of Phoenix in March, 2012.

An Integrated Sense of Self

As the psychic "muscle" of my diabetes consciousness continues to grow, I can't help but embrace the sense of greater self-awareness more and more. I always have the sense of "I have diabetes" in the background, sometimes even in the foreground of my waking consciousness. I do not refer to myself as a "diabetic" because *I Am* not a diabetic. ***I Am** a person who lives in a body that has diabetes.*

As I age, I have grown in wisdom, experience, and understanding to live life as fully as I choose. In my life, diabetes does its own thing, but its guidance and partnership flow from the directed attention of my own thoughts, actions, choices and self-care behaviors. Through meaningful diabetes self-care education, I have learned to think and act as the beta cells that have ceased to function in my body. I use my blood glucose meter, insulin pump, continuous glucose monitor sensor, and amylin injections to serve as my beta cell tools; my consciousness, self knowledge and understanding fill them with intentional directed energy. (In other words, "I" have to do it for my beta cells.) Wherein, that is one of the beauties and blessings of living with diabetes – it is a chronic disease that can be lived with, as long as you know what to do, how to direct the energy and make the choices that are right for you.

I cannot forget who I am, or the fact that I live with diabetes, for even a minute. It is a 24/7 job. I am who I am in my everyday life, and I live, fully integrated, with my diabetes as a body-mind complex. I have a parallel sense of self-knowing at every waking moment. I am constantly vigilant and aware of what is going on in my body, emotions, and thoughts.

Every day, I coordinate the conscious awareness of my diabetes and my self-care actions to partner with my insulin pump, continuous glucose monitor (CGM), and amylin injections to function as a "Pancreas Team" in my body. When I sleep, my pump and CGM watch over me to alert me of the impending dangers of highs and lows. The beeps and buzzes from the pump and CGM alarms serve as "diabetes awakening." They are "reminder tools" that help me focus when I am so absorbed in the day-to-day routines of just plain living and working that I "forget" to remember my self. I have integrated my beloved pump and the CGM into my overall "diabetes consciousness." They are a part of my "sweet life" process, and I cannot live well without them.

Healthy Diabetes Self Concepts

Living with diabetes has shaped my consciousness and directed my life's purpose. As a nurse healer, I teach people how to *be* in their bodies. I often speak to groups of people, many of whom are facing the challenges of living with diabetes. I will ask a group, "How many here are insulin dependent? Raise your hand if you are."

A few hands may timidly rise up.

I ask, "Is that all?" And then, I announce that, "We are *all* insulin dependent whether we have diabetes or not. If we do not have enough insulin working properly in our bodies, it puts us at risk of running out of the life force." This opens the floor for meaningful discussions and teachable moments about the wondrous life-sustaining properties of beta cell functions within the pancreas. I teach that we *all* need sufficient insulin to survive and live a healthy and productive life in this world on all levels of our being. We need to take care of our bodies in order to live as fully embodied spiritual beings in the everyday world.

Even though I now know what the terms "juvenile" and "brittle" signify when used with the term diabetes, I choose *not* to use them when I describe my type 1 diabetes. In other words, I have type 1 diabetes, *period*. I educate my patients and other health care professionals to "call a spade a spade," and use the terms type 1, or type 2 or type 1.5, also known as LADA (Latent Autoimmune Diabetes in Adults), or MODY (Maturity Onset Diabetes of the Young), or gestational diabetes to describe what type of diabetes someone has, because it's important for people to know what type of diabetes they have. It is like knowing your genetic code. Not all diabetes is created equal!

As a nurse healer, my focus is to educate and empower people to make wise decisions for themselves regarding their health and overall well-being. This goes for *everyone*, whether they have diabetes or not. I am not holding out for a "cure" for my diabetes, or anyone else's for that matter. But I do believe that diabetes can be *healed*. Attitudes and lack of knowledge can be improved with meaningful education and loving self-respect, and that's what helps to heal people. I consider my diabetes a blessing and have experienced many diabetes-related healings. My sweet life with diabetes has guided and directed my spirit on the path of life.

Living Life the Way I Want To

I resisted becoming a professional diabetes educator for many years because I did not want to focus my attention on diabetes all the time. There are other dreams and avenues of life and creativity for me to explore and experience. I have always lived fully, in ways beyond my expectations, and my life isn't over

84

yet. But in spite of my best intentions, I can never forget about my sweet life with diabetes. It is always here with me, no matter where I go or what I do.

The journey of self-discovery in being a woman with diabetes continues every single day. I am now pleasantly middle-aged, and have entered the phase of being a Wise Woman. I honor the "Crone" wisdom that comes with living a well-seasoned life. Through pursuing my work as a diabetes educator, I have met some amazing women with diabetes whose friendship, love, and support help to heal and inspire me. I am proud to be affiliated with the national community of DiabetesSisters, establishing PODS (Part of DiabetesSisters) Meet-ups in my area of New York State. Lately, I have been adapting my wardrobe to wear my new favorite colors, orange and golden yellow – the colors of Diabetes Sisterhood!

Living with diabetes has enabled me to see through the eyes of others who live with diabetes and to "walk in their shoes." I really believe that is what makes me an effective CDE with my patients. I understand what they are going through, and I can share real life experiences and practical solutions.

I am not perfect, nor do I have all the answers. I admit that I have my share of sloppy diabetes self-care at times when I do not pay attention to my "diabetes consciousness." But, as long as I can live and function in this body, with fairly decent functional capabilities, I will continue to do so. My spirit-infused diabetes self-consciousness sustains my health, wellness, and self-healing. As long as I have all the necessary beta cell hormone replacements and data generators through a pump, injections, CGMs, and implants – whatever works best – I can and will survive and *be whole*. When the time comes to give up my physical body and surrender into the light body of my soul, I pray to God the Creator that I can cross over quietly and peacefully in my sleep, with my self-awareness and Higher Self consciousness intact.

My husband, Ben, is my best friend and support person. He does not have diabetes, but he honors and lovingly respects the fact that I do. He accepts me for who I am and how I am. Diabetes isn't an issue between us, nor is it a burden for us. It's just a fact of life. We live with it and we deal with whatever comes up. We look forward to growing old together, along with our furry family of eight (yes, eight!) pussycats that live with us.

My widowed mother, Lillian, lives next door so Ben and I can keep an eye on her and be there to assist when needed. With failing eyesight and hearing loss, she is eighty-five years old and slightly frail. She still has a lot of spunk and energy in spite of her age, and continues to teach dance and *tai chi* to senior ladies in her basement dance studio. I observe her for clues to my genetic patterns for aging. She does not have diabetes – my father was the genetic link to type 1 diabetes, as I found out after both he and my aunt, his sister, were also diagnosed with type 1 diabetes – but our bodies are similar. A lifetime of dance practice, therapeutic movement, and exercise goes a long way to preserving physical function as we age. I am so grateful that my mom taught me how to dance at a very early age; we've both kept it up for a lifetime.

It is a full circle between my mom and me – she adapted her life to provide care and assistance for me as a child and youth with diabetes. Now I have adapted my life to provide care and assistance to her in her senior years.

Diabetes has gifted me with *life*, in the fullest sense of what *life* is all about. My sweet life with diabetes has taught me self-discipline. It has enabled me to cultivate love, patience, gratitude, and compassionate sensitivity in relationships with my family, friends, patients, and the greater diabetes community. I also have very strong, loving and healthy partnerships with my health care team and professional colleagues. But, most importantly, I have a strong working relationship within my own consciousness that integrates my everyday life and diabetes self-awareness with my Higher *self* and God, the Creator of All That Is.

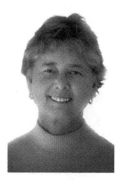

Chapter 8 *by Sally Joy*

There is Life After Kidney Failure

In 1966, at age sixteen, I was diagnosed with type 1 diabetes. I was fortunate to have been diagnosed after the discovery of insulin as, prior to 1921, I would not have survived. I had a two to three day stay in the hospital after I was diagnosed, then I went home.

After my mom brought me home from the hospital, I remember walking into the house and seeing leftover breakfast food, including donuts, on the kitchen table. I felt the straight-jacket of food restrictions wrapping itself around me at that sight! (Now, there are no real food restrictions – you can make adjustments in insulin dosing to accommodate high carbohydrate choices.)

In those early days after my diagnosis, diabetes was rarely discussed. Perhaps it was due to my parents; they completely lacked knowledge about diabetes, and they might have been afraid that I would pre-decease them. Whatever the case, diabetes was never the center of any family conversations and I felt like I was on my own regarding my care.

I guess it really doesn't matter how much my diabetes was discussed. Consider that many of the tools and technology, not to mention the specifics of contemporary diabetes self-management education that we take for granted today wasn't available in 1966. I suspect my brothers, two of whom became doctors, didn't enjoy talking about diabetes because they may have feared that if they had children, their children might end up like me and have type 1 diabetes.

As I look back at the tools, technology, and education I got in 1966, it feels like those were the "dark ages!" Diabetes self-management education was minimal, there was no such thing as home blood glucose monitoring, no insulin pumps or continuous glucose monitors, and carbohydrate counting was practically unheard of. My insulin regimen was very basic: 30 units of NPH (intermediate-acting) insulin once a day. From 1966 until about 1978, I kept up this routine. The results were disastrous, but most of their horrible effects didn't appear until years later.

During my college years and early-mid twenties, I lived a rather carefree lifestyle and rarely visited a doctor. I lived my life without paying much attention to my diabetes. I worked as a house painter (my parents were probably wondering why they sent me to college), managed a greenhouse, sold garden plants and nursery stock, and did maintenance on interior landscape plants.

In my late twenties, I trained to become a dental technician and fabricated gold and porcelain crowns and bridgework. Around this time, I began to suspect that my health might be in decline, so when I moved to Ann Arbor, Michigan, in the late 1970s, I decided I'd better get some help with my diabetes.

In 1978, I was instructed by my doctor to increase my insulin injections to two times per day. Whoa! I thought this must be the beginning of the end – *two* shots per day. I was so uneducated about my diabetes that I didn't realize that taking insulin twice a day could actually improve my blood glucose. This was the first, tiny step on the long road to better diabetes self-care.

Later, I learned about home blood glucose monitoring from my brother, Bill, who was in medical school at the time and doing grand rounds in obstetrics and gynecology. He spoke of pregnant women who monitored their blood sugar to ensure healthy pregnancies. This intrigued me. I had stopped testing my urine for sugar more than a decade earlier. Why perform urine tests when the results were always bad? Besides, testing urine was like reading yesterday's newspaper for the news you wanted right now. I decided that doing my own blood sugar testing might provide a better way to keep track of my diabetes management.

The physician I had been seeing told me that blood sugar testing would not change my life. That was the last time I visited his office. I decided I simply had to try this new technology and was lucky to find a new physician at the University of Michigan who encouraged me to utilize the new home blood glucose monitoring system. A short time later, I discovered a book that provided wonderful coaching on this new technology and how to make it work for me.

While my diabetes management was starting to improve, I married Harry. We met bicycling and he became my most avid supporter and sidekick. He took a real interest in helping me pursue better blood sugar control and assisted when I had low blood sugar reactions. People with diabetes who have a concerned person devoted to them are lucky – I know how lucky I am!

I acquired my first meter in March of 1981. When I began testing, my blood sugar levels were in the 200+ mg/dL to 300+ mg/dL range most of the time. These high blood sugars had occurred for years and were an invitation to later complications. After about six months of blood sugar testing, I saw dramatic improvement; I have been monitoring and fine-tuning my blood sugar control ever since.

Around 2000, I began using an insulin pump, which provided me another level of refinement in my insulin delivery system. However, my first fifteen years of unmanaged diabetes had already taken its toll. In the early 1980s, I began to have retinal (eye) hemorrhages, trouble with *peripheral neuropathy* (lack of feeling in my feet), and ulcers on my feet that would not heal. Here I was, in a relatively new and happy marriage, but I was coming apart at the seams.

Although I got started late in the diabetes management game, when I caught that ball, I ran with it. As well as getting control of my own blood sugar, I was asked to facilitate a Diabetes Support Group that had been started by a nurse who had diabetes. When that nurse left Ann Arbor, a friend with diabetes, Linda, and I took over the Diabetes Support Group and kept it going during the 1980s and 1990s. Here's a sample newspaper announcement: "Semi-Monthly Meeting: Diabetes Support Group. A group for diabetics, people related to diabetics, or those just interested in diabetes. Designed to fill the gap between medical treatment and the realities of living with diabetes. Seasoned veterans share 'trade secrets' with newcomers, including personal accounts of getting through difficult times, new diet regimens, and more."

I realized that discussing ways to cope with diabetes with other people dealing with the same illness was beneficial to me. I also realized that offering a hand-up to others who were having the same difficulties that I was, provided a very strong sense of giving, and it felt good to give. Those of us who attended the Diabetes Support Group shared personal accounts of getting through difficult times. We offered a shoulder to cry on, a pat on the back, and tips for living successfully with diabetes. We explored the concept that "laughter is the best medicine" and often discovered we could laugh about some of our situations while still maintaining our focus on diabetes control. Bottom line: we all learned.

Then came the biggest challenge: in 1985, when I was thirty-five years old, my kidneys failed. My medical team monitored my kidney disease process over several years. At the beginning, when I was asked to bring in a twenty-four hour urine collection – a test to evaluate kidney function – I wasn't sure why. As my ankles continued to expand with fluid retention and kidney disease progressed, I began to learn about the importance of the new tests I was taking and the different medications and dietary changes I was being asked to make.

Even utilizing "delay tactics" (the recommended medicine and diet), my kidney disease progressed. The weeks and months that preceded kidney failure were tough to get through. I had many bouts with nausea and vomiting, had a heart attack induced by fluid overload, and I became weaker and weaker. Looking back, I wasn't sure I would survive.

The good news is that *dialysis* treatments, or a kidney transplant, can maintain your life. Or, as I now tell people, "There is life after kidney failure!" I chose to do *peritoneal* dialysis. Most people think of *hemodialysis* when you say "dialysis." People on *hemodialysis* treatments visit a dialysis facility three times per week and spend about four hours per visit with a machine that pumps their blood through an artificial kidney to remove waste products and extra water – the job your kidneys used to do. But *peritoneal* dialysis is done at home and would be under my control – I liked the sound of that. I was on dialysis for about six months, until I received a kidney transplant. Dialysis wasn't any fun, but it sure beat the alternative of dying at age thirty-five.

When my medical team asked if I wanted to pursue kidney transplantation, I said yes. There are two ways to receive a kidney transplant. One way is to find a living donor. This is a person who matches your blood and tissue type and is healthy enough to donate. I was disappointed to learn that my immediate family members were uneasy about offering to donate to me. As one of my brothers said later, "You weren't such a good risk to bet on and I could just see you getting my kidney and then dying . . . with my kidney!" The other way is to receive a kidney from someone who has died and is a blood and tissue-type match. In the fall of 1985, I was put on the kidney transplant waiting list.

On January 17, 1986, at 2:00 AM, I received a call from the University of Minnesota Hospital saying they had a deceased donor who was a match for me. I jumped on a plane immediately. Later that day, I received my new kidney. The "Gift of Life" is the perfect description for what happened that day. My donor was a seventeen-year-old male who died of suicide.

I wrote "thank you" letters to the family of my donor for several years. Of course, no "thank you" letter can ever explain all the feelings you have – especially knowing I owed my new life to the tragedy another family had to endure. I sent my letters to the organ procurement agency and they forwarded them to the donor family. Then the time came when the letters were returned as undeliverable with no forwarding address.

Not a day goes by that I don't give thanks for the gift I was given. This year, I celebrated my twenty-five-year kidney transplant anniversary.

After my kidney transplant, I started volunteering as a Peer Mentor in the Nephrology Unit at the University of Michigan Hospital. I worked closely with a renal social worker, Erica, and met with other kidney failure patients. Social workers can tell their patients, "there's life after kidney failure," but a picture is worth a thousand words. I would visit with people who felt sick, were scared to death of starting dialysis, and fearful of losing control over their lives. I didn't give medical advice, but was able to "tell my story" and share with them how I was able to manage dialysis treatments and then improve my health even further by receiving a kidney transplant. Since almost half of all kidney failure is caused by diabetes, my Peer Mentor volunteering was like participating in a "roving diabetes support group." I met lots of people facing kidney failure, many with diabetes, and tried to give them a new sense of hope for their future.

I never thought my kidney transplant would last forever. As a matter of fact, at the time I received my transplant, the prevailing wisdom led me to believe that my transplant might last about seven years.

In 1991, I was convinced that I would never see my "golden years," so my husband, Harry, and I decided to rent out our house. I thought, *If I can't have golden years at the end of my life, I am determined to have them right now!* So we bought a pick-up truck and a fifth-wheel travel trailer, and we toured the country for a year. This was a fabulous trip that made me realize I could do more than I thought I could.

When we got back home after a year of touring the country, our finances were depleted. I decided to look for part-time work.

My first job was as a social work technician at a local dialysis facility. There is no shortage of record-keeping and paperwork that renal social workers are responsible for in dialysis facilities. As a social work technician, I did much of the time-consuming paperwork so the social worker could actually do social work! This position worked out well and I stayed for about two years. My next job was part-time at the Renal Network of the Upper Midwest. Again, there was no shortage of paperwork in that office and I helped to keep order.

During my time of Peer Mentoring, working at the dialysis facility, and then at the Renal Network, I had outfitted myself with skills and knowledge. All of it related to chronic kidney disease and kidney failure. These activities enabled me to see kidney care from two sides – the healthcare/business side, and the patient side, which involved people who were often struggling and in need of dialysis and/or kidney transplant. The lesson I learned was that both sides are important.

The National Kidney Foundation of Michigan wanted to get involved in public policy, and hired me to begin their program. I still wonder how that happened. I have a Bachelor of Fine Arts degree from the University of North Carolina (Greensboro) and had no training in government affairs or public policy! What I did have was good logic, decent writing skills, and a passion for issues concerning diabetes, kidney disease and kidney failure. I was eager to share my story and initiate policies that could improve the lives of people with diabetes, chronic kidney disease, and kidney failure, partly because I am 100%

sure that my kidney failure could have been prevented (or at least delayed) with better diabetes management during my early years with diabetes.

I had many excellent role models and "coaches" who helped me gain confidence and perfect my skills as a public policy consultant for the National Kidney Foundation of Michigan. As it turns out, my passion has probably been my most valuable asset.

Diabetes is the leading cause of kidney failure. In my case, type 1 diabetes was not preventable. However, pre-diabetes and type 2 diabetes, which is often caused by obesity and sedentary lifestyles, is now at epidemic proportions. You can connect the dots and see that there will be huge healthcare problems ahead.

I am lucky to work for the National Kidney Foundation of Michigan, an organization that has a mission to prevent kidney disease and kidney failure. This organization develops and implements many disease prevention and disease management programs. My story makes me a credible representative and advocate for their, and my, goals.

Paying for public health programs to support diabetes and kidney disease prevention is a whole 'nother ball game. Much of my advocacy work involves convincing state legislators in Michigan to support public health funding for diabetes and kidney disease prevention programs. Again, I use my story to get their votes.

Working for the Kidney Foundation, I have been able to advocate for public health programs to prevent disease. I have had many meetings with state legislators and have testified many times before the Appropriation Subcommittee for the Department of Community Health in the Michigan House of Representatives and Michigan Senate. In the late 1990s, I helped to get the "Diabetes Cost Reduction Act" passed. This legislation mandates that all health insurers, except "self-insured" employers, cover diabetes education, diabetes testing supplies and diabetes medications.

In 2005 and 2006, I helped to get legislation passed to require GFR (Glomerular Filtration Rate) reporting. The GFR is your kidney score and can be calculated whenever you have a CBC (complete blood count) test. Now, people in Michigan can see their GFR results and talk with their doctor about kidney disease management if their score is too low for their age or is declining too rapidly.

Who would have thought that, in my fifties, I would learn to conquer several computer programs and desktop publishing? I am very proud of an annual "Guide for State Legislators" newsletter that shows how diabetes and kidney disease prevention programs provide value for money invested, improve health, reduce healthcare costs and bring "match dollars" to Michigan. I have organized a Diabetes and Kidney Advocacy Day every year for almost a decade to educate policymakers about the importance of preventing and managing diabetes, chronic kidney disease, and kidney failure.

I also gain support from select legislators by choosing them as "Champions of Hope." The Champions of Hope event is sponsored by the National Kidney Foundation of Michigan and recognizes outstanding state representatives and state senators for their "contributions in healthcare and public policy and providing eternal hope and healing to the citizens of Michigan." It's always good to have champions in the legislature you can call upon when you need help!

Another activity I have adopted within the last ten years is volunteering in a program called the Family Centered Experience at the University of Michigan Medical School. Every two years, I am paired-up with two new medical students and I meet with them during their first and second years in medical school. We get together six or seven times over the two years and they accompany me to one clinic appointment. My role is to teach these students how to see the patient as a whole person and help them understand how living with a chronic disease affects many aspects of your life.

One of my most important messages to these students is that I, the patient, want to be involved in the decision-making about my own disease management. I tell them, "I want to be a part of the team – not a bystander!" I also say that some people with diabetes will choose *not* to participate in their diabetes care. This alarms me, but it is their right and their choice. I urge the students to continue to offer all patients with diabetes involvement in their own care even if they'd rather opt out, with the hope that they will eventually come around. I think a person with diabetes who is a part of his/her own healthcare *team* can have better results in the long run.

Health policy is an issue that has become increasingly important, both at the state and federal levels. I continue to explain to legislators that the huge amounts of money that are spent on healthcare will soon be unsustainable. This is especially true when it comes to kidney failure. The costs for dialysis and kidney transplantation are enormous. I hope I live long enough to see a decrease in diabetes, kidney disease, and kidney failure.

I am at the point now where I am contemplating a semi-retirement from public policy consulting. My passion for preventing kidney disease and kidney failure has not diminished, but my energy level has. Soon I will begin to pass the baton to another, who will continue the advocacy efforts for funding public health programs in order to prevent diabetes and kidney disease. I feel certain that if Michigan, and our nation, do not embrace chronic disease prevention efforts, we will all drown in healthcare costs. Needless to say, I've had my share of healthcare spending. I'm not very proud of that, but the medical care I have received has kept me going.

When I'm not working in our state capitol, I love to garden, swim laps, practice yoga, and walk as much as my legs and feet will allow. Inviting friends for dinner is also one of my nicest pleasures. Meal planning can be a little tricky with diabetes, but I have discovered that if you love to eat (I do!) and you want to feel good (i.e., keep your diabetes under good control), it can be done. I can adapt almost any menu or recipe to be "user friendly" for my diabetes. I have also adopted the custom of having a glass or two of red wine with dinner. What a pleasure from the humble grape.

I didn't invent the phrase, "when you get lemons, make lemonade," but I have tried to make the most of my life with diabetes! Do I wish to come back in my next life without diabetes? Of course. Have I made the most of the hand I was dealt in this life? I hope so.

I often wonder how my life would have turned out if I didn't have diabetes. While I would never wish diabetes on anyone, I must confess, it opened doors that otherwise would not have been there for me. I am grateful to have been able to devote energy and passion to helping people prevent and manage diabetes in order to prevent kidney disease and kidney failure. It's a pleasure to get up in the morning and look forward to going to work.

Website: www.nkfm.org

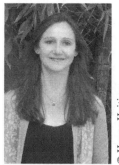

© Hanna Heiting

Chapter 9 *by Zippora Karz*

I Hope You Dance

Dancing was always important to my family. My grandmother Gloria danced a solo act on the Vaudeville circuit, while my mother Ellen studied modern dance at New York's famed Juilliard School and performed many traditional folk dances, including Russian, Romanian, Yugoslavian, Bulgarian, and Israeli. Both danced throughout their lives.

So perhaps it's not surprising to learn that I first learned to dance when I was six years old. At the time, my family lived in Thailand; I remember the beautiful hand and head gestures of the Thai dancers there, so subtle, yet elegant. When we moved back to the United States after my father's Army duties, my mother asked my older sister and I if we would like to take ballet lessons. She said yes, so quite naturally, I said yes as well.

Up to that point, the only ballet I'd seen was on television. I thought the women looked silly with all the pale makeup on their faces, and equally silly acting as if they were having otherworldly experiences. I was not impressed, so I changed the channel. I clearly was not one of those little girls with dreams of becoming a ballerina. Instead, I wanted to be a veterinarian, or perhaps a teacher for the blind and deaf, inspired by the story of Helen Keller.

I didn't acquire my love for dance right away, either. After my first two years of training, I was bored and ready to quit. But the third year of ballet was when you got to take the class from Sheila, the studio's main teacher. I would often peer through the window and watch Sheila teaching the older girls. The way they moved their bodies, their whole *focus*, mesmerized me. I wanted to know what it felt like to be one of those girls, as I knew that something magical was happening in there. I wanted to be a part of whatever it was, which is why I decided that I wouldn't quit.

My teacher, Sheila, understood the technical as well as the artistic demands that are required to be a ballerina. She had always wanted to dance for the great George Balanchine, the genius choreographer who brought ballet to America from Russia, revolutionized the dance world, and founded the New York City Ballet. But Sheila had flat feet and couldn't get *en pointe*, so she put all her passion into teaching.

Her love was infectious and, in time, as my body became stronger, I fell in love with dance, too. The whole experience of moving to music in a trained body was what I wanted to do, but at that point, I still didn't know if I had a future in dance. I was just happy taking classes with Sheila and performing in the end-of-the-year performances at a local high school.

But Sheila knew differently. Sheila believed I had the potential to be a professional ballerina, and that I was suited for George Balanchine's New York City Ballet. Most major ballet companies have schools that train students in the summer and the winter, and the New York City Ballet was no exception. Sheila made sure I auditioned for the New York City Ballet's official school, the School of American Ballet's (SAB) summer program. I received a scholarship twice, first at fourteen years old, and then again at fifteen years old.

After my second summer at the School of American Ballet, the director of the school asked me to stay for the winter program. She told me that if I wanted to become a professional dancer, it was important for me to stay for the winter at my age. But I thought, *Are you crazy? I'm only fifteen years old.* That's why I politely told her that I was going to go home in order to finish high school and then go to college. I'm sure that she thought she'd never see me again.

I flew home to Los Angeles and didn't even tell my mom my news. We didn't have the money for anything like that, and it wasn't something that I wished would happen, so why stress my mom over it? But I told Sheila, because I wanted her to be proud of me. After I took her class, holding my balances longer and lifting my legs higher than before, I hoped she would notice my improvement over the summer. I held back while the other students curtsied and thanked her for the class. Then it was my turn to curtsy.

Sheila asked how the summer had gone. I told her I thought they liked me more this time than the previous year, and then added that they had asked me to stay on as a winter student. Sheila grabbed me by the hand and ran, pulling me through the studio to where my mother waited outside to drive me home. Sheila exclaimed, "You're going!"

It all happened so fast that I didn't have time to think. (I secretly wished someone would say I couldn't go, but that did not happen.) The School of American Ballet awarded me a full scholarship along with some amazing "extras." The scholarship, funded by the Atlantic Richfield Company, was given to just one student each year. In addition to SAB's tuition, the scholarship also covered the tuition for my academic studies at the Professional Children's School (a private school for working child actors, dancers and singers), as well as free lunches in the school cafeteria, $300 per month for living expenses, and two round-trip tickets home during the year.

In 1980, at fifteen years of age, I moved to New York City. It was a big adjustment. At first, I felt totally lost, really missed home, and was on the phone with my mother and younger sister, Romy, every night.

After two weeks, I was told that the director of the school wanted to see me. As I walked to her office, I was worried that they might change their mind about giving me such a generous scholarship. Instead, she told me that I would be moving up to the next level, and that I would now be in the second-highest level.

I was just beginning to make friends, and didn't feel ready to be thrust into a class where most of the other girls were sixteen to eighteen years old. I was an anxious mess and I cried to Romy that I wanted to come home. Even though I loved dancing and I was getting the idea that I was good at it, at that point I didn't have the drive or ambition to be a professional dancer. I still wasn't sure that this was the career I wanted.

Then everything changed. The level I'd been placed in gave me the opportunity to study with the greatest teachers in the world, among them Balanchine's muse. Suzanne Farrell. New York City Ballet company members often took my class, and George Balanchine would randomly appear to pick dancers for the company. I watched Nureyev and Baryshnikov dance alongside the great male dancers of the NYCB in the advanced men's class. Then, there were the performances. Almost every night I watched Peter Martins and Suzanne Farrell, and all of George Balanchine's dancers, grace the stage. I was in awe.

I walked into a world I could never have imagined. Watching and learning from these great artists had a profound impact on me. It seemed that, almost in an instant, I was literally swept up in a world that I had never known existed.

I suddenly felt as if I were being reborn. No longer did I doubt that I belonged there. This had become the only place I wanted to be; my dream now was to dance with the New York City Ballet, for George Balanchine.

Sadly, Balanchine passed away in April of 1983, my third year at SAB. Later that year, I was made an apprentice and, in June of 1984, I was made a full member of the *corps de ballet*. I had just turned eighteen. I went from taking two classes a day and rehearsing for one workshop performance at the end of the year, to taking an hour-and-a-half morning class, rehearsing up to six hours a day, and performing every night, eight performances over the course of a six-day week. When I had prepared for a workshop at SAB, I'd had a month or so to learn a new ballet and many more months to perfect it. Now I was learning, and performing, entire ballets in a matter of days.

What I found was that the sheer excitement of being onstage – the lights, the costumes, the music, the power of the choreography and the energy of the dancers – brought me to a level of energy I never dreamed I had. Although Balanchine was gone, his spirit was alive, due to his ballets, the teachers at SAB, his dancers, and all of those who had worked so closely with him.

My first review was in *Dance* magazine and was written by Joan Acocella, who would go on to become the dance critic for *The New Yorker.* "Zippora Karz, who always looks shiny and clean – as if she were going to a party and her mother just did her braids – glows visibly from whatever corner of the corps she's occupying. One always sees her, hails her, loves her go-for-it eagerness. She seems ready to eat the entire repertoire," Acocella wrote. Even though I was a bit embarrassed to be described as some kind of super-scrubbed Goody Two-shoes, it felt great to be singled out.

In just my second year in the company, Peter Martins, now co-director with Jerome Robbins, singled me out to star as the Sugarplum Fairy in "the Nutcracker." When "young ones" were picked out from the group, it was a very big deal. The reviews hailed my partner, Peter Boal, and me as "potential stars."

Jerome Robbins had come to see my performance in Nutcracker and must have been impressed, as a few weeks later, he chose me to dance a lead in his epic ballet, *The Goldberg Variations*, a role originally created for the great Gelsey Kirkland. Since Balanchine's death, Jerome Robbins (*West Side Story*) was the living genius and master choreographer for the City Ballet, producing amazing works all the time.

I became obsessed with working my body as hard as I could to increase my muscle strength. I wanted to be strong enough and consistent enough to dance leading roles, and to someday become a soloist ballerina.

My third year in the company, Peter Martins chose me to be one of eight up-and-coming dancers to be in his new ballet. I was ecstatic; to have the director choreograph a ballet around you is an incredible honor.

But I was frustrated with the strange things happening in my body. I was thirsty all the time, hungry, dizzy and "spaced out" and couldn't stop urinating. It was the end of a four-month-long winter season, where I had danced all day and performed every night. I was exhausted, and I was under a tremendous amount of pressure with the premiere fast approaching. I thought my symptoms were the result of being burned-out and that I just needed to rest.

I avoided seeing a doctor, convincing myself that I could will myself through my symptoms. But I developed sores under my arms that got so infected

I couldn't lift my arms, and antibiotics did not heal them. It was terribly painful to lift my arms, which ballerinas do a lot, not to mention how unattractive it was. Had it not been for the sores under my arms that threatened my performance, I would not have gone to the doctor and had blood work done.

I was told I had diabetes. My diagnosis was informal and cold, with little information besides all of the horrific things that would happen to my body in the future. I sat in that office and was handed pamphlet after pamphlet about diabetes and its terrifying complications: from heart disease and stroke, to blindness, kidney failure and loss of limbs. As the doctor threw (maybe placed) four different pamphlets about the complications of diabetes in my lap, all I could think about was getting back to the theater in time to get my makeup on so I could perform that evening. I couldn't process the information of the different warnings of what might happen to me in the future. In response to my question of what to do for this "diabetes," the doctor told me that it was okay to eat a piece of cake as long as I did not go overboard and eat the whole thing.

She didn't know me; I didn't trust her. I was a disciplined dancer who was not going to eat cake anyway, especially if I was not supposed to. I didn't have time for more talk, as I had to get back to the theater. She told me to make another appointment so we could discuss the treatment plan. I left the office, both confused and annoyed.

Back at the theatre, I convinced myself that when I got some rest, my blood sugar levels would go back to normal; maybe the blood work was off because of my exhaustion, or it could have been a lab error. I was a twenty-one-year-old aspiring ballerina with the New York City Ballet. A disease people give money to at charity events had nothing to do with me.

I never did make another appointment with that doctor. I was clearly in denial, fueled by the fact that, because of my age, the doctors I had seen initially assumed I had type 2 diabetes. I was put on oral medication. Even though I didn't want to accept it, type 2 diabetes meant I could reverse it. With my dancer's discipline, I set out to perfectly control everything I ate while exercising all day. This actually worked for a time; unbeknownst to me I was still in the "honeymoon phase" of type 1 diabetes.

Everything came crashing down when the honeymoon phase ended. No matter how perfect I was with every morsel of food put into my mouth, I could not keep my blood sugar levels down. Going on insulin felt like the ultimate failure. I hated my body for its inadequacies. I felt hopeless at the thought of how I would juggle shots of insulin with my performance schedule, due to the effect that exercise has on insulin absorption. Every ballet had different stamina requirements. I felt like a human Yo-Yo with blood sugar levels up and down all the time.

The first year I managed my diabetes while taking shots of insulin was extremely difficult, as I tried to maintain tight control (blood sugar levels as close to normal as possible) while performing. I was afraid of the long-term complications, inexperienced with how much insulin to take at any given time before dancing, and unaware of the immediate danger of lows. And I was terrified my directors, Peter Martins and Jerome Robbins, would think that diabetes had changed my dancing and stop calling me to leading roles.

After many severe *hypoglycemic* reactions, often on stage, I realized that my tight control approach was not working. I should have discussed my difficulties with my doctor, but I didn't have the ability back then to talk about it. At this point, I was not talking to anyone, my family included, about my struggles. Everyone knew, but I was not the kind of person who wanted anyone to feel sorry for me, especially when I had no compassion for myself.

Fueled by my desire to run away from my situation, I ran away from my doctor. The new doctor also thought I had type 2 diabetes, like my first two doctors, and took me off insulin. He even told me to stop using my blood glucose meter. He thought the lows on stage were far more dangerous than letting my blood sugars go up a bit. He thought I was being obsessive. Could he have been right?

It's hard for me to understand how I convinced myself it was okay to let my blood sugar levels go high. I was still hoping the whole thing would go away or would reverse itself. I was happy to put the blood glucose meter away and stop my shots.

It didn't take long for my original symptoms to return. My denial was so great, along with my conviction to never go back to shots of insulin, that I never thought to check my blood sugar. I think dancing all day and night, and eating as perfectly as I could, is how I survived with no insulin for almost a year.

But I looked and felt terrible. A dancer needs to feel every part of his or her body, from fingertips to toes. When my blood sugar levels were off, even the slightest bit, I couldn't feel that vital connection. Even though the company still let me dance in the *corps de ballet* every night, there were no leading roles coming my way.

When I finally "woke up" and checked my blood sugar levels, the meter reading would not go that high. It was time to end my denial, take responsibility for my body, and accept my insulin-dependent diabetes.

Educating myself about the disease and how to live and dance with it became my new obsession. I started a balanced insulin program, and began looking and feeling better. I learned not to take too much insulin before I went on stage, thereby avoiding disastrous lows. Ironically, as I learned how to perform every night without experiencing extreme lows, I also psychologically started to question the reality of my situation.

Was this a suitable lifestyle for a person with type 1 diabetes? Maybe I was putting too much pressure on myself? I was exhausted from all the ups and downs with my physiology and from trying so hard to prove I was the same promising dancer I had once been. But I was not the same. Maybe it was time for me to admit I had accomplished a lot, but it was time to find a more suitable lifestyle for a woman with insulin-dependent diabetes?

As much as I wanted to quit dancing, I just could not let myself do it. When I listened to the small voice in my heart, I admitted to myself that if I quit, I would be using diabetes as an excuse. The truth is, I was more tired about wishing I could be the dancer I once was, alive and joyful, than I was tired of diabetes. I had only recently begun to dance on the right insulin regimen, and had not tried it long enough to know what was possible. I did not want to look back with regret, to always wonder, so I had to stay and keep trying.

Nine years after I joined the company (six years after my diagnosis), I was promoted to Soloist Ballerina of the New York City Ballet. I performed with the company another seven years, sixteen years total with the company and thirteen with diabetes. It was not always easy, but I loved every performance and am grateful for every moment I had on stage.

Today, I am a teacher and I stage George Balanchine ballets all over the world. The lesson I have learned about perseverance is one that I now pass on to my students. My message is simple: passion and connection is what motivates us, and gives our lives meaning. If our lives have meaning, we want to feel good. My passion for dance gave me a reason to strive to be healthy. We all experience rejections, we all have failures; the point is to learn from them, to move through them, to take care of our bodies and continue to grow and thrive. To be committed to the process!

Everyone needs to follow a healthy diet and exercise, not just people with diabetes; get enough rest and take care of your emotional health. Find doctors you trust and with whom you are comfortable communicating. Stay connected with your loved ones; I still call my sister Romy every day.

We are only human and diabetes can be difficult, but we have advances that allow us full lives. Today I see insulin as a blessing, giving me life. Throughout my dancing years, I rarely talked about the intricacies of my struggles with diabetes. I wrote my memoir, *The Sugarless Plum*, with the hope of motivating others to take care of their health so that they might live their dreams. We can live full, healthy, passionate lives, and still have diabetes!

Website: www.zipporakarz.com

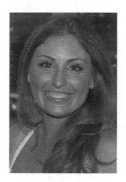

Chapter 10   *by Kelli Kuehne*

Diabetes Fits Me to a Tee

My Diagnosis

I remember walking into the doctor's office when I was ten years old. It was September of 1987; I had just started the fifth grade. My mom (I call her "Momma") was with me, but I was still terrified. I knew something was wrong.

I had gone from being an energetic kid, with a good appetite for food and life, to a "blob." All I wanted to do was sit, drink gallons of water, and go to the bathroom about fifteen times a day. I had lost about six pounds, and that definitely was not normal.

Momma, of course, had noticed the change in me. So there we were, sitting at the doctor's office. I was not happy about it. Momma didn't tell me this at the time, but she had a sneaky suspicion that I was about to be diagnosed with juvenile diabetes. And she was right.

The doctor ordered a urinalysis, and it showed my sugar was really high. He told me I had *diabetes mellitus*.

I looked at Momma and asked, "Am I going to die?"

She calmly said, "No. We will learn all about diabetes and you will be better than okay." Her reaction to my diagnosis was the basis and pillar of why I am able to manage my diabetes, and her reaction spilled over to my father and two older brothers.

I believed her then, and I still do. But I often wonder how I would have managed this in her place. (If my daughter, Morgan, were to receive this diagnosis, would I be as calm, cool and collected as Momma was with me?)

While I was the one diagnosed with diabetes, my family made every sacrifice right along with me. They went through all the trial and error with foods, they checked their blood sugar right along with me, and my dad even stuck himself with a needle so he'd understand my experience as much as possible. My family's self-sacrificing behavior, along with their support, is a major reason why I have been successful in managing diabetes. I am incredibly grateful.

Day One

Newly-diagnosed with juvenile diabetes, I had to immediately meet with an endocrinologist to figure out how I was supposed to manage this disease. He pricked my finger and a strange machine spit out a number – 376 mg/dL. I looked at him and asked, "What does that mean?"

The doctor said, "You will have to take insulin shots for the rest of your life."

I replied, "Okay. That's all?"

He seemed surprised.

I looked at Momma and said, "I can do that."

She replied, "I know."

I was terrified, but it would have been far scarier to know something was wrong, but not know what it was. I almost felt a sense of relief, because we knew I had diabetes, and I could learn to manage the disease and live what everyone kept referring to as a "normal" life.

The doctor went into a long explanation about how I needed to check my blood sugar, keep it within a target range, eat a certain way, and take insulin shots before breakfast and dinner. The list of things to do just kept on coming. (I was ten. My attention span was fifteen seconds.)

I thought at the time, *Okay, I'm out of here.* Not so fast! I still had to get my first shot.

The doctor demonstrated a practice shot on an orange, and then I had to give the orange a shot. Next, it was my turn. I looked at my doctor and said: "I'll do it. This is something I am going to have to do for the rest of my life. I can do this."

He handed me the syringe, coached me through it, and the rest is history.

I look back on it all now and I laugh. I was ten, very confident, and determined. I can't imagine going through the diagnosis and the initial trial and error phase of living with diabetes any other way. I had amazing support from my family and my doctors, but in the end, I was the one who had to live with it. So I started paying attention and taking control of the disease.

Week One

The first week of living with diabetes was a blur. I went from a general practitioner, to an endocrinologist, to a nutritionist. I was told, "Eat this. Don't eat that. Do this. Don't do that." Today, it's no longer so strict; foods and lifestyle fit together.

All of the new information I received was incredibly overwhelming! I was a ten-year-old little girl with so much to learn.

So, I did what many ten-year-olds would do. I grabbed the encyclopedia and looked up "diabetes." That was not a good decision.

I ran down the stairs. At the top of my lungs, I asked my mother,"Why did you lie to me?"

She said, "Kelli. Calm down. What are you in such a tizzy over?"

I replied, "Read this." I pointed to the encyclopedia. "I'm going to die! Or go blind. Or have my toes amputated."

She told me to put the encyclopedia away and breathe. Then she explained that I would live a happy, healthy life if I took care of myself and managed my diabetes. Momma had a way with words. When she laid down the law, you listened. That's what I did, and the encyclopedia didn't make it off the shelf again.

Family Dinner and Sugar-Free Custard

We are all from Texas. Momma is a Southern cook. Everything she fixes is fried. Unfortunately, Southern cooking didn't mesh well with my diabetes. I remember one meal in particular; in fact, everyone in my family remembers this meal twenty-four years later. In hindsight, it was a defining moment for me, and living with diabetes.

Without me knowing, mom and dad told my two brothers, Trip and Hank, whether they liked it or not, they had to eat like me. They didn't have a choice. My parents felt it was important to not alienate me because of my diagnosis.

I don't remember the main part of the meal; none of us do. But we all remember the dessert. Momma whipped up sugar-free vanilla custard. I was pumped because I was going to get dessert. I couldn't wait!

I looked across the table at my dad as he hovered over the custard. I looked to my left at Trip. He wasn't overly thrilled with the custard, but it was going down. I looked next at Hank. He was twirling the custard around with his spoon. That was not surprising, because he was (and still is) a picky eater. Then he asked for Cool Whip. Now, his custard was twice the size of what it was when he started. I looked at Momma, and she was not looking overly impressed with her first attempt at a sugar-free dessert, either.

I decided to give the custard a whirl anyway. I took one bite, looked at my family and said, "No offense Mom . . . but this custard really sucks!" We all cracked up. Unfortunately, Hank had to finish his huge bowl of custard and whipped cream. To this day, none of us will touch custard. In fact, custard still makes me cringe.

Why was this a defining moment? I can never underestimate the impact that my family had on me by making the choice to eat the same way I had to eat.

To some, this may seem insignificant, but to me, it meant I wasn't in the fight against diabetes alone. I had my family's support. I never had to hide how I felt or what I was going through. They always listened. They were always there. They learned all about diabetes, right along with me. That was incredibly empowering.

My Family

My family is loud. We are opinionated. We love each other like crazy. I always say we put the "fun" in dysfunctional. I mean that in the best way!

While I am the youngest of three, my parents never treated me any differently than my brothers. I am blessed that they had the insight to raise us that way. My parents were always adamant that we work hard and give whatever we were doing our best effort. This is extremely relevant, because I applied that same discipline to managing my diabetes.

My mom and dad insisted I become educated about life with diabetes by learning the cause and effect that certain foods have on my blood sugar. The beauty is they did it with me. They had my back one hundred percent. They demanded that I be proactive, so I would never become a victim of diabetes. I continue to live my life in the very same way.

Sports

I was diagnosed with diabetes about the same time I started playing golf with my dad and brothers. At the time, I would never have guessed the significance both events would have on my life!

I was on a sports team for as long as I can remember. I loved running around on the soccer field. I also golfed, played tennis, and basketball. Fortunately, my passion for sports didn't die because of my diagnosis. I just had to learn to adjust.

For example, I had to learn what to eat so I could maintain my blood sugar levels on the field during an hour-long soccer game. My teammates would bring me Life Savers® and orange wedges as they substituted in and out of the game. I also had to learn what to eat to play eighteen holes of golf and maintain my blood sugar levels. Momma would make two peanut butter sandwiches and cut them into four squares, so I could eat a square at a time every hole or two.

People with diabetes have to make adjustments and figure out what works for them. It isn't the same for everyone. The only way to learn is through trial and error.

Before I started playing golf, I was a competitive tennis player. I loved it. In the summer of 1988, Momma and I traveled across the country to tennis events, while my dad traveled the country with Trip and Hank for junior golf tournaments. One day, when we were all together on a break from competitions, I looked at my brothers and said: "Heck with this. I'm going to play golf so the family can travel together."

My brothers and I spent the next seven years playing competitive golf and traveling the world. Trip started college at Arizona State University, at Tempe, Arizona, and then transferred to Oklahoma State University at Stillwater, Oklahoma, on a golf scholarship. Hank went to Oklahoma State, and then transferred to Southern Methodist University at Dallas, Texas. I went to the University of Texas at Austin. That is when and where my life and health dramatically changed for the better.

My Trainer and My Doctor at the University of Texas

Tina Bonci was, and still is, the head women's athletic trainer at the University of Texas at Austin. She also had juvenile diabetes, or as it's now called, type 1 diabetes. When I first met her, I was eighteen-years-old and thought I had it all figured out. Tina took time to talk to me about living with diabetes during my first few days at the University of Texas. I more or less blew her off. How dumb! I am not proud of doing that.

A few weeks later, I became more interested in what she had to say. When she showed me her insulin pump, I thought it was incredible. I had never seen anything like it. She explained how it worked, and showed me what it looked like up close. I thought about it for several days, and then we talked again.

Ultimately, she made an appointment for me with a local endocrinologist – Dr. Tom Blevins. He turned my world upside down and inside out. He educated me in a way that was inspiring. He made me want to learn even more about living successfully with diabetes.

Both Tina and Dr. Blevins have been incredibly influential in my life. They gave me a new base for understanding life with diabetes. I switched to an insulin pump a year later. It was 1998, eleven years after being diagnosed with diabetes.

The Device That Changed My World: My Animas® Insulin Pump

My ability to control my diabetes was always good, but Tina and Dr. Blevins pushed me to make it even better by switching to an insulin pump, and I accepted the challenge.

The insulin pump was ideal for me. I had just finished a less than spectacular rookie year on the Ladies Professional Golf Association (LPGA) Tour. I had been on a combined regimen of short- and long-acting insulin shots for more than eleven years. The pump was a difficult (but welcome) change, which gave me the tightest possible control of my blood sugar levels.

I now wear a One Touch Ping Animas® insulin pump, and many people ask me about it. In my opinion, the only way to show someone exactly how the pump works is to give them a very honest and hands-on experience. So I show people where my pump is attached. My site is in my abdomen. I unhook the quick release and let people see what point-one (.1) of a milliliter looks like coming out of my infusion set.

The reaction I get from people with diabetes is surprise, typically followed by the question, "Where do I get one?" I could talk about my insulin pump and the benefits of it forever, but people want to see how it actually works and I can completely understand. Tina did the same thing for me thirteen years ago when I asked her the same question, and it changed my life.

Once people understand the flexibility and consistency that the insulin pump offers, it becomes a viable option for managing diabetes. If my "show and tell" approach inspires someone to pursue better maintenance, then I have achieved my goal of encouraging healthy living with diabetes.

The idea of an insulin pump is to provide insulin which is unavailable in a person with type 1 diabetes due to a malfunctioning pancreas. When you eat, your blood sugar level goes up. The goal is to offset the elevation of your blood sugar by taking a bolus of insulin that offsets the spike in blood sugar levels. The rest of the day, you are getting a basal rate, which is a set amount per hour, based on your body's insulin needs.

The amazing part about the pump is it is more or less self-regulating. It's much easier to see the patterns of your blood sugar levels and make the necessary adjustments based on those patterns. My Animas® pump takes a lot of the guesswork out of it for me and gives me the opportunity to enjoy a more flexible schedule. I still check my blood sugar levels throughout the day, but I always wear my pump. It gives me huge peace of mind.

Golf

All I wanted to do was chase my two big brothers around. Whatever they did, I did. That's how I ended up choosing golf. I played competitive soccer and basketball, but soon realized that, although I always enjoyed playing on a sports team, I enjoyed one-on-one competition better. (Shocking, I know.)

I competed on the American Junior Golf Association (AJGA) Tour from ages fourteen to seventeen years old. The AJGA was a junior national tour that helped develop me into the player I became.

I won seven events on the AJGA Tour. In 1994, I won the United States Junior Girls Championship. In 1995, I won the US Women's Amateur Championship. In 1996, I represented the United States of America in the Curtis Cup (which is the US versus Europe) and the World Cup (which is the US versus the world), and won the Women's British Amateur Championship in England. I also won the US Women's Amateur Championship again in 1996. I was the only golfer in history to win the US Junior, the US Amateur, the British Amateur and the US Amateur in consecutive years. To be completely honest, I thought winning all of those events at the time was normal. I know it sounds crazy, but it is true.

I received the Southwest Conference Player of the Year honors and was a First Team All-American in 1996 during my freshman year at The University of Texas. I also had the honor of being inducted into the Texas Sports Hall of Fame.

I turned professional in the fall of 1996. I was nineteen years old. It was the next logical step for me with my golf career. I have been incredibly blessed to do something I love for so long. I was blessed with the opportunity to play, travel, see the world and meet some amazing people along the way.

Professional golf also gave me the platform to make a difference in people's lives who live with diabetes. In 1998, I was named a National Spokesperson for the Juvenile Diabetes Research Foundation (JDRF). That role has given me a greater sense of accomplishment than golf ever has. My family, and a few friends, used to run a golf fundraiser in Texas called "Teeing It Up for the Cure to Diabetes." We raised over $2.4 million dollars for the JDRF. That is something that I am so proud of!

I played on the LPGA Tour for thirteen years. I earned over $2.2 million dollars in prize money and had one victory, the 1999 LPGA Corning Classic. I also had the opportunity to represent the United States, twice, in the Solheim Cup in 2002 and 2003. It was nerve-wracking, but probably the most pressure – and most fun – I have ever had playing professional golf.

I heard a statistic the other day: the odds of becoming a professional golfer are one in 250,000. Not succeeding in the professional golf world was never an option for me. I am not one to tolerate excuses, which is why diabetes was never an excuse for me to not follow my dreams.

I express that to all of the young kids who I meet and work with. Golf is not easy; it's not supposed to be. Learning to live with diabetes is not easy, either; it's a choice. Some days will go flawlessly, while others will be a challenge. In my opinion, the challenge is what makes it all worthwhile.

My Husband and Step-Daughter

I am a very lucky woman. I am married to an amazing man, Paul Doremus. We have a two-year-old daughter, Morgan, who I've helped to raise since she was six weeks old. While she is technically my step-daughter, I consider her my own child.

I remember the day I met my husband. We talked about anything and everything, and we haven't stopped talking. I have always felt it is important to be very upfront about living with diabetes. Paul understood.

I explained my daily rigors of living with diabetes, checking my blood sugar levels, my dietary needs, my golf game, and my hectic schedule. None of it scared him away; instead, he embraced it. He made learning about and understanding diabetes a priority. He went through "the initiation" of finger sticks at my side. His support and eagerness to learn about living with diabetes has been incredible.

Morgan, my daughter, knows every day that I check my blood sugar and take my insulin. She watches me like a hawk. I explain to her that I have to do these things to be, and stay, healthy. She seems to understand. When I give Morgan her vitamins in the morning, she says, "This is my vitamin. I want two, so I can be healthy like mommy." I laugh, but it does make me proud. My husband and I believe it is our responsibility to educate our daughter and make her aware of healthy living.

Life's Scorecard

Today, I really don't remember my life before diabetes. After I was diagnosed, I remember being the kid who everyone wanted to be near at birthday parties, because I never ate the icing off of my piece of cake. My plate was a free-for-all, because every other kid at the party wanted my icing.

That wasn't ever awkward for me; instead, it was empowering. It may sound odd to some, but it is my perspective. Life is what you make of it.

For me, living with diabetes has been a blessing. I truly believe it, because I have had the opportunity of a lifetime to meet and have a profound impact on so many lives. That has been incredibly gratifying.

Learning to live with diabetes takes time. It also takes a work ethic and unusual discipline. There are days my blood sugar levels are ideal. There are also days when I struggle to keep it within a desired range. Luckily, those days are few and far between.

I honestly believe I was chosen to have insulin-dependent diabetes. I believe God only gives you what He knows you can handle, and that there is a plan for us all. For me, it is to overcome and thrive while living with diabetes, and to pass my knowledge on.

My good friend, Tina Bonci, has given me so much good advice and guidance throughout the years. When I was eighteen years old, she said something to me that I've never forgotten. She said, "Whatever you keep doing will get easier the longer you do it. It's not that what you're doing has changed its nature; it's that your ability to do it increases the longer you work at it."

I was smart enough to listen to her advice, and it's now how I live my life. Some days, I am great at it, other days, not so much. However, when I have days that I struggle, I can still hear Momma's voice saying, "You can do this. You are going to be better than okay."

Your golf scorecard only contains numbers that determine how great or how bad you are at the game. You can't draw pictures or write comments in the scorecard box describing the elements, or the course conditions, or any handicaps you faced indicating you played better than your score. So in a way, it doesn't tell the whole story of what you did.

On life's scorecard, you have the opportunity to create whatever picture you can imagine, with diabetes or without, and then make it a reality. How you choose to live with diabetes is up to you. So take it one day at a time, color outside the lines, create something incredibly beautiful and make it a Hell of a ride!!!

Website: www.kellikuehne.com

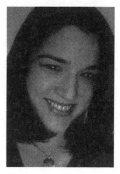

Chapter 11   *by Kelly Kunik*

Life's Glass - Perpetually Half Full

My chapter is dedicated to my amazing mother Marjory Kunik, who passed away after a brief illness during the week my chapter was due. Mom was the person who taught me to view life's glass as being perpetually half-full instead of half-empty. She is the one who taught me that whether your "pancreas is broken" or not, life goes on. And it's up to you to make the best of what you're given and live the best life you possibly can. She is the reason for both my positive attitude and my green eyes. Thanks for all your life lessons and love, mom – I love you!

I see my life's "glass" as being perpetually half-full. Perhaps this is because I was diagnosed on Halloween – I kid you not – and I've now spent more years with diabetes (thirty-four) than I did without it.

I don't remember too much of what my world was like before my diagnosis. I have faint memories of ice-cold, green bottles of Sprite® for thirty-five cents from an antique blue Pepsi® machine after tap class on Saturday afternoons. I also remember going to Sunday matinees and downing the occasional "Pixy Stix®." But, if the truth is to be told, I was more of a "Fun Dip™" girl myself. (Fun Dip™ was similar to Pixy Stix®, but sold in small pouches, rather than paper or plastic straws. It generally consisted of three packets of flavored, colored sugar. It was intended to be consumed by licking the sticks and using the moistened stick to collect some of the sugar.) I also remember eating popsicles on the beach, followed by playing "Cut The Cake" with the stick afterwards. Those sugar-filled visions dance in my head from time to time, but memories of my life, in general, before my diagnosis is fuzzy, to say the least.

Right before I was diagnosed, I remember losing an incredible amount of weight and being thirsty all the time. I also remember my older sister, Debbie, asking me to urinate on something called "Tes-Tape®." I remember my whole family sitting around the kitchen table and saying, "Kelly's sugar is off the charts." I knew exactly what that meant, because my father and two older sisters all had type 1 diabetes.

It was Halloween morning, so I begged my parents to wait until the next day to take me to the hospital, because I didn't want to miss dressing up for Halloween. They didn't wait, of course; they drove me right up to Children's Hospital in Philadelphia. A nurse, dressed up as a clown, was the person who told me that I definitely had diabetes.

Life after my diabetes diagnosis was both similar and different, all rolled up into one, and I remember it much more vividly. My parents forced me to forge on and move ahead, so my "normal" became different from that of my friends. Both parents told me in the hospital that diabetes would now be a part of my life for a very long time and that, in order to live a great life, I needed to accept that fact. So I did.

Life for a person with diabetes was *so* different back in the late 1970s. We had urine testing instead of blood glucose testing; the "diabetic diet" was strict and there was no such thing as carbohydrate counting or insulin pumps. Taking your "reading" meant testing your urine, which was disgusting and involved fuzzy blue Clinitest™ tablets, glass droppers and tubes that would burn your fingertips in thirty seconds flat. It was like having a science lab set up in your very own bathroom – a science lab that was inaccurate and disgusting, but a science lab nonetheless.

The American Diabetes Association diet was hung on the kitchen wall, next to the phone and right under my seat at the kitchen table. My mother counted grapes in groups of twelve and only bought small bananas, which she would then cut in half before putting a banana on my plate. She measured low fat milk and glasses of orange, grape and apple juice precisely. (To this day, I've never poured more than a quarter of a glass of orange juice in one sitting.) At dinner, we had little "baby-sized" baked potatoes instead of full-sized spuds, accompanied by lots of green stuff – much to my dismay.

Diet chocolate pudding and diet cherry Jell-O® became my desserts *du jour*. There were three types of diet sodas on the market, and everything tasty was off limits. TaB® and diet Pepsi® became my "go to" staples, and I drank more diet soda than any third-grader should. My needles would be boiled nightly (even though they were disposable) and sat right next to the tea kettle.

I realized early on that insulin was both life-saving and expensive, and that insulin was both precious and a necessary evil. Every urine reading was

118

written down in a big red log book, then reported back to my endocrinologist every Friday afternoon.

Life went on – diabetes diagnosis or not – and my parents refused to let life stop or pass me by. I took gymnastics three times a week, tap dancing class on Saturday mornings, singing lessons on Monday afternoons, and went to the math tutor on Thursday evenings. I slept over at friends' houses, was involved in community theater, had birthday parties with real cake (we always had real cake on special occasions) not the disgusting, "diabetic-friendly" cakes. Easter baskets were filled with books, sugar-free chewing gum, Star Wars toys, Barbie memorabilia, Bonnie Bell cosmetics, and a new stuffed animal to love. I still made the best Halloween costumes and I "*Trick-Or–Treated*" with a vengeance! (My parents were smart enough to allow me to put the chocolate candy aside for special occasions.)

My parents explained to me what would happen if I didn't eat my snack during class in great detail. They talked about the consequences of skipping that snack: I could pass out, have to go to the hospital, or have a seizure; they sugarcoated nothing – no pun intended.

My older sister, Debbie, showed me those diabetes "worst case" realities at a very young age, as she passed away when I was in college. She was only thirty-five, and died due to complications from type 1 diabetes. For most of my childhood, Debbie truly suffered due to her diabetes; her life was closer to those "worst case scenarios" than not. Debbie was fourteen years older than me and had been diagnosed in the late 1960s, when diabetes management lacked any sense of flexibility. I think about her often, and wish things had been different for her.

Because of Debbie, I ate my snacks in class every day and never skipped them. Also, I never hid the fact that I was a person with diabetes - I didn't want to pass out in the gutter and have my friends misunderstand the reason why. My friends and classmates, for the most part, were great about my diabetes. And the ones who weren't? I'd learn many years later that, nine times out of ten, their behavior had nothing to do with my diabetes or what was going on in my life. Instead, it had *everything* to do with what was happening in their lives.

Blood glucose meters became available when I was in the fifth or sixth grade, but they were incredibly expensive, took three minutes to calibrate, and another three minutes to calculate your blood sugar. Plus, there was *nothing* convenient – or subtle – about them. Blood glucose meters were the size of a brick, and weighed about as much!

There was no easy way to carry a glucose meter on the sly. Back then, meters made school backpacks heavy, and they wouldn't fit in a handbag, no matter how hard you tried to shove it in there. I'm not proud of the fact that I fought my parents regarding our family's communal glucose meter.

I want to be perfectly clear: I made plenty of diabetes mistakes growing up. (I still make mistakes, for that matter.) I was a far cry from the perfect "Person with Diabetes" (PWD), especially as a teen, and many of my diabetes "mistakes" were intentional. I was a teenager, and I knew "*everything*." I worked hard to be "normal," and wanted to be like everyone else. In college, I studied diligently, and I continued to work just as diligently to fit in, regardless of my "broken pancreas."

But "normal" with a broken pancreas meant I took my insulin with me to class and injected whenever and wherever I was, be it in the library, the cafeteria or at a *kegger* (party). I always made sure that I had food with me just in case of a low blood sugar reaction. But did I test my blood sugar as often as I should have? No, I did not. Did I do what I shouldn't and ignore my diabetes? Yeah, there were times I did. (I'm extremely lucky to have lived through all that.) Over time, I learned that I was an imperfect PWD, and my life – both personally and professionally – went on.

Shortly after college, I learned not to hate my diabetes. As a matter of fact, I learned to accept my diabetes and work with it, rather than against it. I actually started to embrace my diabetes, because I came to realize that, like it or not, my diabetes was a part of me. It was like being left-handed, or having green eyes. If I hated my diabetes and all that it encompassed, I'd end up hating myself. I refused to do that. I deserved better, and I knew it!

Instead, I found a great endocrinologist and a great Certified Diabetes Educator and learned to *own my diabetes* (at least, most of the time), so that my diabetes wouldn't control me anymore.

Diabetes forced me to speak up for myself, even when I didn't feel like it, which, in turn, gave me a sense of self-confidence that has stuck with me over the years. Diabetes has given me a highly developed sense of humor and empathy, both of which come in handy in my work, not to mention my life. I've learned not only to speak up for myself (because if I don't, who will?), but also to enjoy the totality of my life, including my diabetes. I also take great solace in the fact that my diabetes has given me some interesting stories to tell at dinner parties.

Do I still get frustrated and annoyed with my diabetes? *You bet I do!* I'll be the first to admit that there are days when my blood sugar refuses to go down (or up) and my diabetes literally drives me nuts. There also are days when I do everything right and my diabetes *still* somehow manages to "one-up me," just because it can. But I acknowledge those moments of diabetes craziness, and blog about it on my "diabetesaliciousness" diabetes blog. I also take the time to laugh out loud whenever possible, regardless of my "diabetes insanity." The same goes for shedding a tear, because sometimes, I just need to cry!

I'm the first to admit my diabetes mistakes. For example, I've miscalculated carbohydrates. I've forgotten extra pump batteries, and also forgotten to bolus for a meal. I've also over-bolused for meals, big time, and had to eat like a horse so my blood sugar wouldn't go low. I've had the dubious "pleasure" of having my insulin pump tubing get wrapped around doorknobs, and the pain of ripping out my pump infusion sets at the most inappropriate and intimate of moments.

In case these mishaps aren't enough for you, here's a few more that have occurred over the years. I've dashed off to work *sans* my insulin pump, and had to turn the car around ASAP in order to retrieve it. And then, I've had to call my boss and let him know I was going to be late and the (diabetes) reason why. I've inadvertently smashed my last full bottle of insulin on the bathroom floor and had to run to the pharmacy for a refill; then have my insurance deny payment because I refilled my prescription too early. Perhaps the oddest of all, I've been met with looks of surprise and fright after yelling, "Darn it! I'm high!" in the middle of a crowded restaurant after testing my blood sugar.

So as you've seen, I've definitely had many diabetes moments where I couldn't help but ask, "*WHY ME?*" Of course, those moments are then followed inexorably by the question, "*WHY NOT ME?*" (In those moments, when all is right in my diabetes world, I'm incredibly happy and grateful; I thank my diabetes out loud for behaving.)

Over the years, I've come to realize that every single person in the world has a different view of "normal." Their "normal" is different from yours, and your "normal" is different than mine, whether you have diabetes or not. The bottom line is that *everybody* has something; nobody's "normal" is the same, and that's perfectly okay. So I embrace *all* that is normal in my life, and in my diabetes world, and learn from those moments, which is why I continue to view life's glass as half-full.

There will be some days in both life and diabetes that will be harder than others. On occasion, my "glass" will lean more toward the empty line, rather than the full; those are the days that will be the toughest. But, luckily for me, life's glass is never half-empty for long. I know that there will be plenty of days when my glass will overflow with laughter and joy, and I want you to realize that, diabetes or not, life is what you make of it, so make your life an amazing one!

Website: www.Diabetesaliciousness.com
Website: www.Diabetesalicious.com

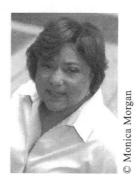

© Monica Morgan

Chapter 12   *by Jacquie Lewis-Kemp, MPP*

Diabetes and Organ Transplant: No Limit on My Lifestyle

Diabetes – How it All Started

My maternal grandparents often took me on fishing trips. It was our chance to eat pizza and enjoy the outdoors – not to mention catch that day's dinner. This time, we had gone to a place in Canada with a long dock, a place where many people went to fish.

My grandmother always packed for "just in case." She had extra food, a jug of water to drink, and another with which to wash our hands. She had extra clothes for all of us, including shoes. She had learned the importance of this after my cousin fell in the river; my grandfather saved her. While my grandmother had a complete change of clothes for my cousin, she only had a towel for Granddaddy.

Our fishing trips were so frequent that it was my grandmother who first noticed my symptoms of diabetes. We were fishing on the dock when I had to go to the bathroom really badly. My grandmother walked me back up the dock to use the public restroom. Knowing she had a jug of water, I asked for a cup of it. She obliged, and then we returned to the fishing spot.

No sooner had I gotten back to my chair that I had to go to the bathroom again. So my grandmother escorted me, again, up the dock to the public restroom. And again, I was thirsty, so my grandmother gave me more water. She decided to take the water out to where we were fishing so that all of us could enjoy it, but out of the entire jug, Granddaddy may have had a cup. I remember drinking the ice dry in the two-gallon thermos. We also made several more trips to the bathroom.

When we returned home, Granny told my mom that she'd better get me checked out by the doctor because we didn't fish a lick. This is why, at my two-month-old baby brother's next appointment with the doctor, my mom asked the doctor to check me out. He drew a random sample of blood (not a fasting blood sugar test); the result showed that my blood sugar tested very high, way out of the normal range. Mom's two-month-old son was fine, but her daughter had diabetes.

It was August 1969, when I was seven years old, that I was diagnosed with diabetes. Nobody else in my family had "juvenile diabetes." At that time, children with diabetes were routinely hospitalized after their diagnosis and were taught to give themselves insulin and learned how to manage the disease. My recollection of my first night at the hospital is visions of bright chrome and white porcelain. My father always told me stories at bedtime, and in the hospital, he also told me one until I drifted off to sleep. The first night, I woke up after he left, jumped from my bed and ran screaming down the halls. The nurses quieted me and put me back to bed, promising that he would return in the morning. The only place that I had spent the night away from home, prior to the hospital stay, was at my grandparents' house.

The doctors spent time not only regulating my blood sugar, but also teaching me how to manage my diabetes. The most important thing they taught me was how to give myself a shot. The days in the hospital got better as they explained that I would learn to give myself shots. (That sounded like I would be a doctor!) Sure enough, before I left the hospital, I knew how to give myself an insulin shot and my parents knew how to sterilize my glass syringes and draw up my insulin.

I missed two months of the second grade, and I couldn't wait to tell my friends that I'd been away at "medical training" and could give myself a shot – not just once, but every day. I remember my parents reassured me that I could manage my health by living and eating properly. Whenever I asked, "What should I be when I grow up?" both my parents would always answer, "Whatever you want to be, as long as it is something you enjoy. You can do whatever you want, as long as you work hard at it." It's amazing: I still believe that advice, forty years later.

Growing Up with Type 1 Diabetes

Managing diabetes with the best that 1970s technology had to offer was a challenge. Diabetes was managed by urine sugar testing because there were no home blood glucose meters available yet. We used Tes-Tape®, which when dipped in urine, either remained yellow if you had no sugar in your urine, turned slightly green if you had trace amounts, or turned darker greens for moderate to high sugar levels. It was a formidable task to urinate on a 2" x ¼" strip of tape without making a mess all over your hands – and if I touched the test area, the sweat on my hands would react with the tape and cause the test to falsely read higher.

As a child, I went to a camp where all the children had diabetes. Before each meal, we had to test our urine and report it to the counselor, who then recorded it and turned it into the medical staff at camp. The doctors, nurses, and dietitians used it to determine what your insulin doses should be. If you couldn't urinate before a meal, you couldn't eat until you did. (There is not much worse to eat than cold, camp mashed potatoes, scooped out in half-cup scoops.) The camp experience was important. The normal camp activities proved that I could do anything while living with diabetes. Being with other children who had diabetes showed me that I wasn't alone on this journey.

I went to the doctor every six months. My blood sugar was monitored, and the doctor reviewed my log of urine sugar readings, food, and activity levels at different times of the day. Then, based upon urine sugar trends, the doctor prescribed my insulin dosage to take each day until my next visit.

Insulin was different then, too. Long before today's Humulin®, (which is synthesized in a special, non-disease-producing laboratory strain of *E. coli* bacteria that has been genetically altered to produce human insulin), insulin was made from beef and pork pancreases. At that time, there were two different strengths of insulin: U-40 and U-80. If a person took a dose of 40 units or less they were prescribed U-40 insulin and U-40 syringes. Likewise, if a person took more than 40 units, they used U-80 insulin and U-80 syringes.

To complicate matters even more, before plastic disposable syringes, I was sent home from the hospital with a glass syringe that my mother had to boil every morning in order to sterilize it. There was nothing more painful than drawing up the proper dosage, assembling the disposable needle into the syringe, and then injecting it into my thigh, only to have the residue from boiling the glass syringe cause the plunger to get stuck – while still in my thigh! No matter how hard I pushed the plunger, the insulin wouldn't go in. I'd have to withdraw it, push to check the plunger, replace the disposable needle and draw up more insulin, then stick myself again. Sometimes this happened due to the low technology of the needle rather than the residue from the water. There was no such thing as microfine needles in 1969. They were long needles, and they hurt!

Sleepovers required special consideration, too. Mom's rule was that I left my friend's house early to come home and take my insulin, and perhaps I could return if they weren't serving pancakes (which required syrup that I couldn't eat) for breakfast.

Because the taste of artificial sweeteners was so awful in the late 1960s and 1970s, I often opted to eliminate certain foods from my diet rather than ruin a meal with a sugarless alternative. For instance, sugarless candy tasted like cough drops, so I didn't eat candy unless it had sugar and I was cheating on my diet. Sugarless syrup tasted awful, too, so I didn't eat pancakes, waffles, or French toast. For a long time, sugar-free soda came in only two varieties: cola and lemon-lime. I'd rather drink water than endure the awful taste of saccharine in the sodas. Even as I got older, rather than use artificial sweeteners in my coffee or tea, I would rather drink them black.

As a kid, the one thing that made life with diabetes worth living were "Hog-Wild Days." My doctor allowed his patients with diabetes to choose three days out of the year when we could eat anything we wanted. When one of those days hit, hog-wild is what it was! I would eat pancakes with chocolate chips, ice cream and whipped cream for breakfast, candy and chips for lunch and a fast food milkshake for dinner.

On those days, the doctor prescribed extra insulin and my mother monitored me closely. I always chose Halloween as one of those days, so I could eat as much candy as I wanted (as much as my mother would allow) and Easter because there was always chocolate in the Easter basket for my brother. I could never get enough of the bacon the men of the church cooked after the Easter Sunday sunrise service. And, of course, I chose Christmas to enjoy all the holiday desserts.

When I was about thirteen years old (in the seventh grade), my blood sugar went haywire because of my changing hormone levels. I was hospitalized for a week to adjust my insulin regimen. (In the 1970s, it was customary to hospitalize people with diabetes to adjust their insulin dosing.) Remember, there was no such thing as home blood glucose meters. Patients with diabetes kept a log of urine sugar test results measured four times a day.

My doctor scheduled appointments every six months to measure my actual blood sugar. Based upon the trends set by the urine sugar and the fasting blood sugar, taken at the visit, the doctor would adjust my insulin dose. This required quite a bit of calculating from the doctor, since urine sugar values reflected blood sugar history; determining insulin requirements, at best, was a *guesstimate*.

Also in the 1970s, U-100 insulin and U-100 syringes were developed. This was an advance from the previous U-40 and U-80 insulin and syringes. These "universal" U-100 insulin and syringes seemed to be the best thing since sliced bread, at least for those of us who took 100 units of insulin or less. I don't know of anyone who took more than (or even close to) 100 units. The other advancement was that they were completely disposable. No more boiling syringes!

The other change during that hospital visit was that the doctors said I needed to take two shots per day. This news didn't mean that my diabetes had somehow worsened, but was due to a change in diabetes management philosophy. Doctors realized that multiple insulin injections could mimic a functioning pancreas by dispensing insulin when needed, not all at once, thereby yielding better blood sugar control.

In my particular case, what this meant was taking my shot and eating a snack before and after school sports. There was no way I was giving up cheerleading, so I carried the insulin, syringes and a snack to school.

I got used to managing my diabetes, and I remained active. I even wrote an article while in high school for the local newspaper called "Diabetes: Just An Inconvenience." At that time in my life, I felt pretty proud of myself – I was managing my diabetes and being a regular kid. As a young child, I knew what the *islets of Langerhans* were (the insulin producing cells of the pancreas) long before today's development of islet cell transplants.

My parents also became educated about diabetes. Doctors were careful to teach us about the long-term complications of diabetes along with prevention techniques. I remember ranking the complications in order of what I believed to be the least to the most severe. I had heard that a distant cousin had diabetes, and as the old folks said, "He had it so bad that he had to have a leg amputated." As visible of a handicap as that was, I figured an amputation wouldn't kill me – so that was my first choice of complications (if I had to have any). I didn't count neuropathy, because a little tingling in my hands and feet couldn't really count as a complication. Next on the list was *retinopathy*, or in its extreme form, blindness. While blindness, too, is a terrible complication, it wouldn't kill me either. I ranked kidney disease as the worst possible thing that could happen. I could live with at least one kidney. But if they both failed, I could die.

As a part of my medical regimen, the doctors monitored how much protein I was spilling in my urine. To measure the amount of protein, doctors periodically ordered a twenty-four hour urinalysis. That test called for me to urinate into a jug for an entire twenty-four hour period. When you have good, working kidneys, lots of urine is excreted in twenty-four hours – especially if you have high blood sugar with the symptoms of constant thirst and frequent urination. The nurse issued a "hat" (a medical term for a receptacle to urinate into) with a spout and a plastic jug to store the urine in. The urine had to be stored in a cool place and they would prefer that you refrigerated it. In the winter, that was no problem because it could be stored in the garage or outside

127

in the snow. It was more of a challenge in the summer to keep it cool, and not have Jell-O® taste like urine because it happened to be right next to the urine collection container in the refrigerator.

Life with diabetes was a little different than what most kids experienced, but not much. We just had to create a bypass around some situations. Having supportive and involved parents was critical, and I credit my parents most for my ability to function without using diabetes as an excuse. My mother put her career on hold for almost five years and allowed herself time to understand diabetes. She first learned how to boil my syringes and, to my chagrin, she also became proficient at baking desserts with artificial sweeteners, like "Apple Brown Betty," an apple pie-like dessert. Yuck!

My father participated in helping me to understand and manage my diabetes as well. While my mom taught me more of the day-to-day procedures, my dad helped me more with conceptualizing my diabetes and taught me how to live my life with it. At the combative age of thirteen, I was sick of diabetes and taking shots twice a day. My father sat down next to me, in short pants, and drew up water into an insulin syringe. I saw what he was about to do and I said, "Dad, you don't have to".

My dad answered, "If you can do it, then I can do it." And he proceeded to give himself an injection of water.

An Adult with Type 1 Diabetes

I attended college at the University of Michigan, where I graduated with a double major in Political Science and Communications and then I earned a Masters in Public Policy – all in five years. It didn't seem like a big deal. I simply decided upon a major, and then, when I looked at the balance of my transcript, found that I had enough credits for another major if I simply went back and took the prerequisites. Graduate school was an extension of career planning that I began during summer as a sophomore. Given the opportunity to combine my senior year of undergraduate study with my first year of graduate work, I made my way through a full load of twenty-one credit hours in one term and sixteen credits in the other.

I now realize why it didn't seem like such a big deal, and I credit diabetes for that realization. Working hard and planning ahead was always necessary to prevent *hyperglycemia* and *hypoglycemia* (high and low blood sugar, respectively). So working hard and planning ahead became my way of doing things overall. Why shouldn't this extend into my college studies? Not only did I learn how to be prepared for my diabetes management, but that understanding of "being prepared" was also useful for managing my studies, and later to manage working and raising a family. After school, I went to work for my father in his automotive supplier manufacturing plant. I worked for my dad for eight years. I felt like I understood most things, but knew that I didn't know everything. But I couldn't have asked for a better supervisor than my Daddy. He knew that he could trust me to hold his confidence and have the company's best interest at heart, always. With that trust, came the responsibility to make a difference.

After eight years of working for my father, he died suddenly, leaving a big hole in the company he founded and in my heart. But this is where my diabetes training helped me to focus, work hard, and get through my grief. I stepped into my father's role as Chief Executive Officer (CEO) and ran his company for an additional ten years.

I married, and two years later, we had a son. Well, given my high-risk pregnancy that required me to see my high-risk obstetrician twice a week, from the time that I was eleven weeks pregnant until I delivered at eight months (thirty-six weeks), I think it is safe to say that *I had* a son, with support from my husband.

Being pregnant made me manage my diabetes in a completely different way. Early in my pregnancy, my doctor ordered tests to check my baseline status regarding long-term complications. I had already seen a retina specialist, just prior to my wedding, who treated my *retinopathy* with laser surgery (a procedure where laser light is focused on the damaged retina to seal leaking retinal blood vessels) and a vitrectomy (a procedure where blood is removed from the center of the eye (vitreous)).

I also was seen by a cardiologist, a nephrologist, and a gastroenterologist. My doctor wanted to know what he was dealing with when it got down to the final hours of delivery. All the blood sugar testing, logs, and doctor's visits are examples of how hard work, focus, and planning yielded a positive outcome. A very carefully orchestrated Cesarean section delivery (C-section) produced a 7 pound 11 ounce baby boy. My son is now a college athlete.

Long-term Complications

In addition to the retinopathy that occurred just before my wedding, I also suffered kidney failure as a result of my diabetes. My bout with kidney failure, dialysis and ultimately a kidney transplant was tough and grueling. But, fortunately for me, dialysis only lasted for seven months, before my younger brother offered to donate his left kidney. That's when the transplant process began.

I was evaluated by a social worker, who not only considered my state of mind and family support situation, but also my insurance and my ability to pay for the transplant. They also evaluated my ability to pay for post-transplant medication, which I would need to take for the rest of my life. I was then interviewed by several medical professionals, who also assessed whether I was a compliant patient – in other words, they wanted to know if I would follow the regimen as prescribed in order to protect my new kidney, or if I would fall into habits that would jeopardize my new kidney, like drinking alcohol to excess, smoking, or not taking my medication. The physical tests included an EKG, a cardiac stress test, a chest X-ray and regular gynecological tests, as well as clearance from my dentist, who made sure my dental work was complete and my teeth were without any decay. With green lights in all these categories, I was cleared for surgery.

My brother went into surgery first. I was overcome with emotion that my little brother, someone I had beaten up when we were kids (yet always loved and protected), was about to give me his left kidney and save my life.

After a few hours, it was my turn. I got dressed as I had so many times before with my eye surgery, my C-section, my laparoscopy, and my catheter for dialysis. My abdomen looked like a National Football League playbook. I knew the routine: get hooked up to the IV, take a little oral indigestion medicine, and then a hit from the IV of "feel good." The next trick for me was to try to remember the last thing I saw before "lights out."

During my pre-transplant screening, doctors were careful to describe my transplant as "treatment" for my kidney failure. It was not a *cure*, because in the beginning, there is as much as a twenty percent chance of my body rejecting the transplanted kidney. In fact, they said that acute rejection was likely within the first five years of the transplant and that I should plan on it. And so, I started the rest of my life with a new regimen of immunosuppressant medications and a different set of metrics to monitor.

After the kidney transplant, doctors told me that the best thing to preserve my kidney would be a pancreas transplant. A pancreas transplant would mean that my blood sugar would be normal. The pancreas transplant would not only preserve my new kidney, but stop the progression of other long-term complications of diabetes like retinopathy or neuropathy.

The pancreas is a more delicate organ than the kidney; therefore the transplant is more difficult. To me, what was appealing about the prospect of a pancreas transplant was that, if successful, I would no longer have to deal with the aggravation of either low blood sugar problems or high blood sugar issues, nor would I have to have such an involved maintenance schedule in order to remain healthy. I knew that, if the transplant worked, I would have more time to care for my son and to concentrate on re-establishing my career without the burden of managing my diabetes.

That prospect would have been exciting, except I wouldn't allow myself to look across the river and imagine what life would be like with a functioning pancreas. I also was afraid of setting myself up, only to become disappointed if the transplant didn't work or I was unable to obtain one.

I returned to the transplant team and was completely re-evaluated, just like I was a brand-new prospective transplant patient. After that, I was officially listed on the pancreas transplant list. On May 30, 2002, I received a pancreas transplant.

I lived with diabetes for thirty-two years, from the time I was seven years old. To all of a sudden have what I referred to as an "automatic pancreas," was something I needed to get used to. So many people, myself included, thought that a pancreas transplant would be liberating – I would be free, never again having to take a shot of insulin, free to eat what I wanted (something I'd greatly looked forward to), and much more. But instead, I could feel my blood sugar raising and dropping.

The first thing that I noticed was that my morning blood sugar levels always felt like I was having a low blood sugar reaction. So I would always eat as soon as I woke up. Doctors explained that my new pancreas was surgically connected directly to my large intestine. This sent insulin straight to my bloodstream rather than through my liver, as the insulin was routed with my native pancreas. Because the insulin goes directly into the bloodstream and doesn't receive some glucose from my liver, my morning blood sugar levels are lower than the normal range.

The doctors suggested that I do nothing. My *hypoglycemic* symptoms would adjust to what is now my new normal blood sugar. It took awhile, but I refrained from eating immediately after getting out of bed. Sure enough, my morning fasting blood sugar normalized at about 77 mg/dL and I no longer had *hypoglycemic* symptoms.

I tested my new, "automatic pancreas." After I ate a piece of chocolate, or after a high carbohydrate meal, I would test my blood sugar to see if it had gone up to 300 mg/dL, like it used to do. But it consistently measured at or about 200 mg/dL, which is normal, for a person without diabetes, after eating a high carbohydrate meal.

As time went on, my husband remarked about how my skin looked better and that my feet were no longer cold. My dentist described how much healthier my gums were. The pancreas transplant really had improved my overall health.

When I tell people that I had a pancreas transplant, many ask, "So you don't have diabetes anymore?" I correct them by explaining that first and foremost, my transplants are a treatment for my chronic kidney disease and my diabetes, *not a cure*. A serious rejection episode could end the life of my transplanted pancreas and send me right back to insulin injections; likewise, a rejection of my transplanted kidney could send me back to dialysis.

Another reason that I still have diabetes is that my body lived with thirty-two years of elevated blood sugar levels, which caused some irreversible long-term complications. My *retinopathy* deteriorated to blindness in my right eye because of CMV virus (*cytomegalovirus*) that wasn't caught in time. Because my body is immunosuppressed, it could not fight the virus (nor can it destroy my transplanted organs).

While my daily medical regimen has changed from insulin injections and glucose testing to a fist full of anti-rejection drugs, I still pay attention to what I eat and count nutritional values as I was taught. I grew up not liking sugar-free sweeteners and soda, so after my pancreas transplant, I decided I wasn't going to start consuming high fructose corn syrup.

Recent years have found me conducting seminars about healthy ways to manage diabetes, promoting organ donation, writing a weekly blog on my Website (listed at the end of this chapter), and promoting my book, *Blessed Assurance: Success Despite the Odds*. My book is an inspirational story and includes tips for living life with diabetes, rather than *limiting* life because of diabetes.

When I looked at all that I was able to accomplish while living with diabetes, and examined the likely causes for the confidence to have been a thirty-one-year-old woman with diabetes, African-American, wife, mother, and CEO of a manufacturing company, I realized that for me, diabetes changed from being an obstacle to a motivator for success. I wrote my book, in part, because I wanted more people with diabetes to learn how to use this diagnosis as a motivator.

Now that our son is in college, my husband and I are returning to the life we had before the hectic life of raising a child. A full life is a happy life, and my intent is to make it as happy as I can. So I take on as many projects as I can effectively handle. I volunteer for the Juvenile Diabetes Research Foundation, the American Diabetes Association, "Gift of Life", the National Kidney Foundation and the University of Michigan Transplant Center.

The chronic illness that I understand and live with is diabetes. I've learned that the keys to living a healthy and successful life with diabetes are hard work, focus, and planning ahead. I don't let diabetes – or organ transplantation – limit my lifestyle!

Website: www.jlewiskemp.com

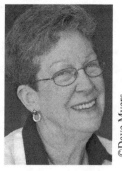
©Dave Myers,
Images Today and Beyond

Chapter 13   *by Joan McGinnis, RN, MSN, CDE*

Diabetes Advocacy: Self-Knowledge to Community Education

My Beginning, without Diabetes

I was born the second of six children, in the medium-sized city of Toledo, Ohio. We had all the usual childhood illnesses, usually all of us being ill at the same time, and survived all of them.

While my parents were well-educated for the time, they were barely making ends meet financially. My mom, a Registered Nurse, worked part-time when she could while I was young, and began working full-time for an obstetrician-gynecologist's office, to help bring in income, when I was nine years old. My mom was a survivor, having lost her mother at the age of two, then living in an orphanage for about five years until her father remarried. My dad had a Bachelor's degree in philosophy, and intended to go to medical school before the economy crashed in 1933. He became a salesman instead, working on commission.

We had a happy and close family, but we did undergo emotionally difficult times: my younger sister became mentally challenged after an ear infection, thought to be due to meningitis. She became a ward of the state at the age of six-and-a-half, as my parents were not able to manage her and provide for her needs. I had been responsible for significant parts of her care, and her absence was difficult for all of us.

In 1961, my father died following a heart attack at age fifty-three. He lived just past my high school graduation. I was very close to my dad, and was not able to grieve.

I needed to get a job and was unable to go to college, as I had planned. I went to work as a file clerk in the Radiology Department of a hospital, where I fell in love with the medical world, and decided I would like to become a nurse. My mom was supportive. I worked during my free time and managed to get some scholarship money for nursing school.

Our family had its share of type 1 diabetes. In 1964, my younger brother was diagnosed when he was seventeen years old. I was in nursing school at the time. At eighteen years old, he left home and got married. He had multiple difficulties with his marriage, job, finances, and a baby, in addition to caring for his diabetes. He experienced frequent low blood sugar reactions.

In 1965, I became interested in obtaining a Bachelor's Degree in Nursing and worked full-time as a coronary care nurse, a head nurse, and attended college part-time for five years. During this time, my second brother developed type 1 diabetes at age twenty-three, after finishing his tour in the United States Navy, then going to junior college. He also exhibited low blood sugar reactions at many family events. I used to think my brothers with diabetes just did not know how to eat and I spent lots of time trying to teach them. They listened to what I taught them, but were living on their own without "male culinary skills."

In 1970, I moved to Saint Louis, Missouri, and finished my Bachelor's degree in Nursing with the help of a scholarship. Over the next few years, I continued to pursue a Master's Degree in Nursing, all the while working part-time in Barnes Hospital's Coronary Care Unit, or teaching at St. Luke's School of Nursing. I knew that I had to be able to support myself, looking at my mom's experience. I met and married my husband, who had a PhD in Philosophy, when I completed my Bachelor's Degree in January of 1972.

The early years of family life were wonderful and we had our first daughter, Sara, in 1974 while I was in graduate school in Medical-Surgical Nursing at St. Louis University. My husband was working at St. Louis University as Director of Academic Advising, and I began working there as a Nursing Faculty Member when my Master's Degree was completed. When our first daughter was born, I decreased to part-time teaching. My husband and I worked on different campuses, had one car, and lived well in a second story apartment.

Our second daughter, Kathryn, was born in 1977. Our lives were very busy and full.

Around this time, my third brother was diagnosed, at age thirty, with type 1 diabetes. I was very upset, on his behalf, as he was my baby brother.

I went to visit him two months after he was diagnosed, and it seemed like I "caught diabetes" while I was there. (Not really – diabetes isn't contagious!) I was up late, talking with him and his wife and drinking tons of coffee. I was so thirsty; nothing quenched my thirst. I was frequently urinating as well, all evening long.

When I arrived home to my place of residence in St. Louis, I went and bought some Tes-Tape® to check my urine. It was full of sugar. I was flabbergasted, but it explained my thirst!

Reaction to Diagnosis

I did not accept the idea, at all, that I had diabetes, despite having three brothers with type 1 diabetes, the positive result of the Tes-Tape® sample, and the knowledge I possessed of physiology due to my nursing education and experience. My thoughts went something like this:

I am a nurse with a lot of experience dealing with others, who are very sick. I feel fine, though admittedly thirsty and frequently urinating, but fine, really . . . maybe there was a mistake in the urine test?

Perhaps the test result was due to some other physical problem, which I did not know about; maybe something worse than diabetes?

I do not have time for an illness. I am a busy mother and I work part-time as a clinical instructor. Diabetes is a disease other people get, not me!

Besides, if you are a nurse, you didn't get these things. I don't know any other health professional who has diabetes!

It's not fair for me to get this! Look at my brothers, who always have low blood sugar reactions. I cannot be a nurse and put up with confusion due to low blood sugar!

Of course, I had all the classic symptoms of diabetes, the "polys": polydipsia (*great thirst*), polyuria (*great urination*), and polyphagia (*great hunger*). But I thought it must be something else. I did agree that I needed to see a doctor to get this resolved – but it couldn't be diabetes!

I was not depressed, because I didn't believe it was diabetes. But my husband was depressed about it, even though he didn't ordinarily talk much about illness; he used to get queasy getting a shot.

I received a recommendation to see an internist. My blood sugar was in the high 200s mg/dL and he told me to go on a 1200 calorie a day diet and exercise. At that time, I probably was consuming 2800-3000 calories on many days, and hadn't run since the sixth month of my first pregnancy. So, I started to run daily for two months and followed the diet. I lost ten pounds and went back to the doctor. My blood sugar was fine – he told me it was "a fluke", just like I thought it was. He said I could eat again and exercise less, and I did.

137

When I returned in another month, my blood sugar was 240 mg/dL and this time I had absolutely no symptoms. (Perhaps I had been in the "honeymoon period" and this accounted for the normal blood sugar reading at the previous appointment?) So I went back on the diet and exercise regimen.

My husband and I decided to have a weekend away from the babies and were going to go a short distance from our town to enjoy a great weekend. After we arrived, I checked my urine for sugar, as I was now doing regularly, and found a lot of sugar in my urine again. I checked for ketones in the urine, as well, and had moderate ketones. I knew ketones could be serious!

I contacted my doctor, who told me to enjoy the weekend and forget about it, but we came home the next day. I was very aware from that moment on that I had type 1 diabetes. But the doctor was not concerned, nor did he recommend that I get help to deal with this disease. But I had to do something, which is why I went to see the doctor the following day. He recommended a *sulfonylurea* – an oral medication – but I refused and said I wanted insulin. (In 1978, you did not usually challenge your doctor. But I knew that, at the time, it was thought that *sulfonylureas* could cause early heart disease in people with diabetes.)

The doctor agreed to prescribe NPH insulin, 10 units a day, and told me to increase it a few units every few days if I still had sugar in the urine test. Taking a shot was not difficult for me, in any way, except psychologically. I had given thousands of injections to others.

Three months later, I happened to see my doctor in the hospital where I was a Clinical Instructor for student nurses. He noted I had lost a lot of weight, was not looking well, and that I looked angry. I replied that I was angry about having diabetes and that I had lost twenty-seven pounds. He asked how much insulin I was taking. I said twenty units. I could not bring myself to go beyond the number *twenty* on the syringe – in my mind, it would mean that I really had diabetes. I felt like I was a total failure and was doing something wrong if twenty units did not cure me.

I went in to see him the next day, and he asked me to take thirty units. He told me that I would gain back some weight, but that I would need to take more insulin. He also told me that since I knew the diet, I would not need to see a dietitian. Even though I did know the diet, I had much difficulty actually following the diet! I decided to see a dietitian on my own. That was a big help to me, as I was able to discuss my personal challenges with the diet and get her advice.

Early Days with Diabetes

Once I got up to about thirty-five units of NPH insulin daily, I stopped worrying about the diabetes and was back to being a Mom and a wife. I was working, and I enjoyed my life more. I gained back ten to fifteen pounds quickly. I could get through the day without worrying so much about the future. But I still would have some low blood sugar reactions on clinical days with students; I carried food with me always, eating more than I needed to prevent lows.

I felt depressed when emptying my coffee can of syringes, as I realized that my diabetes would not go away. I remember teaching my first daughter, still very young, how to call 9-1-1, in case I didn't wake up if I took a nap. I know that I was sometimes irritable to my husband and children and (while I had no way to check my blood sugar) I felt it was due to high blood sugars. Eating out became very difficult, because of trying to decide the proper amount of food to eat, which made my life very un-spontaneous. But, at that time, I knew nothing about how diabetes was affecting me, as there were no blood glucose meters and no A1C test to evaluate your average blood sugar.

My worst experience was developing the Asian flu in 1983, after five years with diabetes. I had never missed a day of work in my life, nor was I ever really sick. While I had the flu, I was nauseated, kept vomiting, and had diarrhea for four days. When I was unable to stand up and go to work, I called my doctor. He told me to come to the emergency room. I said I was a nurse and I was not going to the emergency room. I asked him what I could do to help myself. He told me to drink fluids and call back if I wasn't feeling better.

The next morning, I awoke with labored breathing – which I knew was a sign of *diabetic ketoacidosis* (DKA). I recognized the symptom immediately from caring for patients with DKA in the Intensive Care Unit (ICU). Then I went to stand on the bathroom scale. I had lost four pounds in a couple of days and was very dehydrated. I immediately went to the emergency room; my blood sugar was very high and my body was severely dehydrated. I knew that dehydration could cause serious harm to other organs in my body, which would be deprived of fluid. They gave me fluid intravenously and then lots of insulin to help me recover.

While hospitalized, an endocrinologist came to see me, with his medical residents following behind. He told me my diabetes was out of control. I was insulted, distressed, angry, and embarrassed! Here I was, a professional nurse, and I was just as sick as all the people I had cared for in the ICU. This was the beginning of "Joan's Revolution." I realized my life was just like my diabetes – when my diabetes was out of control, so was my life. I knew I could not control either one totally, but there were things I could do to prevent either from being totally out of control.

Even though this was a very negative experience for me, it was the beginning of my career as a diabetes educator. If I had known something to prevent myself from getting that sick, I would never be sick again. I realized that those who did not understand what I knew as a nurse would be in a much worse situation than me, and I began to understand why all the patients who I had cared for in the ICU put their diabetes at serious risk whenever they were sick. This inspired me to create the "Guidelines for Sick Days," which is now a part of all diabetes education. I knew that all people with diabetes needed considerable education in order to decrease their risk of hospitalization by taking early action when sick.

The Revolution Period

One of the endocrinologists at St. Louis University Hospital sent me to an outpatient colleague. The endocrinologist visit was very helpful; he understood immediately what all of my problems were with regards to high and low blood sugars, and how to evaluate my diabetes control. He told me blood glucose meters were going to be available to patients in St. Louis as a result of a nationwide research study called the Diabetes Control and Complications Trial (DCCT). I bought my first blood glucose meter that week. My endocrinologist also divided my one shot of insulin a day into two shots: morning and evening. And, he added faster-acting insulin at mealtimes, which greatly improved my diabetes control.

One of the endocrinologists at St. Louis University asked me to join the team of interested professionals to develop a diabetes education program. As a member of this team, I attended a seminar on the DCCT at Washington University to hear what they were learning from the study. All of the panelists on the patient presentation had diabetes and most were on insulin pumps (a newer method of insulin delivery with continuous subcutaneous insulin infusion) and had experienced at least one episode of a severe low blood sugar reaction, which required the assistance of another person to help them recover. I was greatly concerned about this.

The team I joined, with Doctors Stewart Albert, Marla Bernbaum, Alan Silverberg, and Dr. Coy Fitch, was planning to expand diabetes care at St. Louis University Hospital and Clinics. They were a committed team of doctors who cared about their patients.

Joan's Revolution

I spent every minute I could finding out everything there was to know about insulin, diabetes, and its complications with a team of endocrinology physicians. Funded by the National Institute of Diabetes and Digestive and Kidney Diseases, the DCCT had been set up with type 1 diabetes patients to compare the effects of standard control of blood glucose versus intensive control on the complications of diabetes. My husband was very supportive of my "revolution," which included gaining new knowledge, new responsibility, and a newer approach to diabetes care. He was eager for me to be in excellent health in the future.

My knowledge base and resources became vast, and I joined the local diabetes educators group in St. Louis, one of the first chapters of the American Association of Diabetes Educators (AADE). I volunteered in the endocrinology clinic for diabetes education for three to four years, armed with an assessment form that would provide a basis for excellent diabetes self-management education. Dr. Stewart Albert helped me to become the diabetes educator that I am today.

Attending that workshop instilled in me the hope that the future of diabetes was much brighter than I had imagined. I began to focus on two new projects: 1) improving my own personal diabetes self-care, and 2) developing an approach to determine what concerns people with diabetes need help with. This has served me well and was based on my own experiences of denial, embarrassment, and knowledge-seeking behavior. I wanted to help improve the communication and assertiveness needed for a better patient-physician relationship.

My Daughter's Diagnosis

A paying position for a diabetes educator became available in the Department of Endocrinology, and I applied for a joint appointment to the School of Medicine and The School of Nursing. I was the first person to have such a position, and felt a strong responsibility to ensure that any other diabetes educators who followed me would be able to have an excellent role model to base their joint appointments on. I made a commitment to try this full-time position for two years. I would be working full-time for the first time in years with two bosses.

The week after I started the position, my husband diagnosed our thirteen-year-old daughter with type 1 diabetes. Almost crying, he mentioned her weight loss, thirst and frequent urination to me. I knew he was correct. I made an appointment with a pediatric endocrinologist for her on the following weekend day, so I would not miss work. After I did so, I realized I was again in denial and called to get her into the clinic the next day. She refused to let me check her blood sugar, but I managed to talk her into it by morning. Based on my blood glucose meter reading of 300 mg/dL, she was admitted to the hospital for a couple of days.

I was depressed for about three weeks. At this point, I was very conversant with the pediatric endocrinologist and felt comfortable making suggestions for my daughter's insulin timing as she got older. My daughter's type 1 diabetes actually increased my knowledge about pediatric diabetes. My daughter felt

141

pretty comfortable with her endocrinologist, who definitely believed that parents and children should learn everything there is to know about diabetes. Of course, at this time, all type 1 diabetes patients were taught to do home blood glucose monitoring, and were given guidelines for adjusting insulin dosing at mealtimes.

Becoming a Certified Diabetes Educator

I passed the Certified Diabetes Educator exam in 1989 and, together with the endocrinologists at the University, devised a Diabetes Education Program for the St. Louis University Hospital and Outpatient Clinic. For years, I was an officer and committee chairperson for the local AADE chapter, called Saint Louis Association of Diabetes Educators (SLADE), going to annual conventions and obtaining every continuing education credit available to me. My challenge was how to make that knowledge available to people with diabetes, so that they could understand more and pursue what they needed as soon as possible after diagnosis. I also served on the State of Missouri Diabetes Education Advisory Committee. I developed the skills necessary to educate visually-impaired persons with diabetes, due to the mentoring of one of the endocrinologists in our department, who had diabetes and vision loss.

While I was interested in the concept of insulin pumps, I was thinking that I might become completely obsessed with diabetes if I used the newest method of insulin delivery. Other people with diabetes, who I met at the annual conventions, would ask me when I was going to start on the pump. I decided against it at the time, partly based on the DCCT panelists on pumps, who had reported that they had all experienced low blood sugar reactions that they could not treat themselves. I assumed, at that time, that the pump may have been the reason, which I later learned was not true.

Later Years with Diabetes

I quit teaching nursing (while I retained my faculty position as an Adjunct Professor) and decided to devote more time to diabetes education. I worked for a private endocrinologist one day per week, in addition to working part-time in the university position. I loved providing diabetes education to people who were eager to learn. I worked very hard on three aspects of diabetes care, including:

1. obtaining Medicare insurance coverage for blood glucose monitoring strips for persons with type 2 diabetes (finally a Federal law by 1998).
2. reimbursement for diabetes education by diabetes educators through insurance companies, the only known revenue source at the time.
3. developing and working to identify, through a Diabetes Committee at the hospital level, where policy and procedure could be initiated to provide the best and safest patient care for persons with diabetes who were hospitalized.

At the same time, in the private endocrinology practice, I worked on getting recognition, through the American Diabetes Association (ADA), for the Diabetes Education Program there. We had a few patients on insulin pumps at the private endocrinology practice. I became very interested in insulin pumps as a source of better blood sugar control, which was evident in the blood sugar records and A1C reports for these people. At that time, I started using an insulin pump. Together with one of the endocrinologists at the university, we learned how to do pump training, and how to get patients to feel comfortable getting diabetes education to improve their lives.

After I was on the pump for two weeks, I knew that I would never choose to be without it, knowing I could now have a more normal life. The year prior to my own pump initiation, I joined a group of patients to learn the skill of carbohydrate counting. Under the supervision of a dietitian, Silvia Carnes, RD, CDE, we furthered our understanding of the role of diet in controlling diabetes and how to lose weight safely. Silvia was an excellent dietitian, willing to try new ideas, which helped my transition to insulin pump therapy.

Bypass Surgery

I left the university position as a Diabetes Educator and increased my hours in the private practice for the next ten years. The position there was much more challenging, and I was encouraged to use all of my abilities by the Director of the Clinic, Jonathan Bortz, MD. We had a collaborative practice agreement which helped me develop my abilities as a clinician, caring for patients on intensive insulin therapy and insulin pump therapy, and new insulin therapies, as well as innovative blood glucose monitoring systems on the Internet. A new technology for people with diabetes, a continuous glucose sensor, was then available and we began using it to help people anticipate when their blood sugar levels might be trending low or high and how to combat that. While working there, at the Bortz Diabetes Control Center, with an interdisciplinary team of endocrinologists, along with a dietitian, clinical psychologist, cardiologist, vascular specialist, retinal specialist and podiatrist all under one roof for a period of time, we made some significant improvements in the lives of people with diabetes.

Personally, while working there, I needed to have bypass surgery in 1998, due to a significant blockage (but no damage to my heart). I needed a stent in 2009, which brought to light again how important education and communication with your physicians can be. I learned again how important it is to ask the appropriate questions to make your hospitalization for surgery easier. My family – father, mother, and four brothers – all had coronary artery disease, and my three brothers with type 1 diabetes all had heart surgery, albeit at a younger age than me.

Since I had the bypass surgery, I walk five to six days a week with my best friend, who has been a significant source of support. I recognized that her encouragement and belief in me was helpful in facing every annual eye exam, every surgery (I have had a few – heart, tendons, and cataracts), lab test, and doctor visits for heart, feet, endocrinology and primary care.

Sadly, the position at the Bortz Center ended in 2003. I then chose another route for patient education.

Community Diabetes Education Programs

I began a new era of private practice to cover the transition for our Bortz patients on the pump to new endocrinologists or primary care physicians. My daughters were grown and I had a completely new interest in diabetes and public health for the increasing masses of people developing type 2 diabetes. I developed a new diabetes support group at an underserved clinic in the city: Community Health In Partnership Services (CHIPS) over a year's time with key personnel there. I wrote a diabetes education curriculum (called diabetes@work) for the St. Louis Diabetes Coalition and the State of Missouri and presented it to the Board of the Coalition.

They endorsed it, and with another colleague, Eric Armbrecht, PhD, who I had previously worked with at the Bortz Diabetes Control Center, developed the program with an interdisciplinary team to deliver to employers, for their employees, over a twelve-week lunch hour delivery. Cindy Merrins MS, RD, CDE, Board Certified in Diabetes, helped me implement the nutritional content throughout the twelve weeks.

Our first program in 2004 was delivered multiple times to different employer groups, demonstrating that education was effective in lowering A1C. In this first program, I initiated an incentive system for participants to attend classes and to complete assignments; they received chances to win a flat screen television. The assignments provided valuable feedback and helped to develop a rapport. That rapport was enhanced by email communication with participants, which allowed for personal one-on-one interaction, as well as group interaction. Group interaction was vital, as it provided an opportunity for people to hear how others interacted with physicians and healthcare providers, and helped to put their own relationships in perspective, which they could then analyze objectively.

I became the Director of Education for the St. Louis Diabetes Coalition in 2006, allowing for education through small and large community workshops, diabetes@work program implementation, radio interviews, and support group presentations in the community. I had lots of experience doing presentations for the AADE, both locally at our SLADE chapter, and nationally at the ADA, National Business Health Coalition, and Public Health meetings.

During the last several years, I have mentored some health professionals in diabetes education, in order to replace myself in the community as I near retirement. I also initiated a DIVA Diabetics mentoring/support group, for women only, with type 1 diabetes, ages eighteen to thirty, which meets monthly at the local Juvenile Diabetes Research Foundation (JDRF) office. Women in this age group are dealing with relationship issues, marriage, pregnancy, education, and employment concerns, in addition to coping with a diagnosis of type 1 diabetes. Many are also struggling to decide which insulin delivery method to choose.

Over the last twenty-five-plus years, I have been privileged to know some of the finest people in diabetes care, including my own endocrinologist, Dr. Garry Tobin, at Washington University Diabetes Center and my boss, Dr. Eric Armbrecht, who is a public health expert, a statistician, a researcher, and an excellent motivational speaker. Together, we have worked on evolving new ideas and approaches for the future of diabetes care and diabetes education. The current St. Louis Diabetes Coalition project, called "KICK Diabetes", provides diabetes education by a Certified Diabetes Educator, at a location close to the participants' homes or work in St. Louis City or County. Education is provided at no cost (supported by a regional health grant) to individuals who have not had access to it and need it. The diabetes educators on this project were especially chosen to provide the very best in diabetes self-management skills.

My Life Has Been Sweet

My life has not been without difficulty and challenge. Growing up, I handled a lot of responsibility as the oldest girl in the family, which endowed me with cooking, cleaning, and child care skills. In some ways, it prepared me for diabetes – especially related to the need for planning, flexibility and discipline. I did not develop my diabetes until a year after my third pregnancy, when our second child was born. Our daughters were beautiful gifts to our lives.

Deciding to ensure that my daughter, who also has type 1 diabetes, had a life without unnecessary limitations was one of the reasons my life has been so good. I never told her what she had to do, but by living as simply and carefully as I did, she learned about assertiveness and self-management skills. Ultimately, she was able to do the same as her sister (who does not have diabetes), choosing to have a meaningful career, get a good education, get married, and most recently, have a healthy baby. My husband, daughters, sons-in-law, and my grandchildren are close and very supportive of what I do and I appreciate their roles in my life.

I also have been blessed to work with medical professionals who have given me good advice and encouragement, both professionally and personally, so that I can make the most of the resources I possess. Accepting my diabetes and learning everything I could about diabetes enabled me to manage my own diabetes in a much better way.

Through my own early experiences, in a time when diabetes education was not available, to newly diagnosed people, I learned how important it was to become assertive in the management of my own diabetes care. At some point, in becoming a diabetes educator, I found my niche in life, helping people with diabetes adjust to living with this chronic illness, and I really loved doing that.

Becoming a Certified Diabetes Educator encouraged me to be a good role model. I found it rewarding to reach out to people with diabetes, challenge some (when I saw they could handle it), and to give positive reinforcement for the efforts of people coping with diabetes.

My professional life has allowed me to share my successes. I feel that the role of the diabetes educator, as an advocate for people with diabetes, provides important information that can teach and model self-management skills, so individuals can assume responsibility for their own healthcare. Helping to ensure competency, the diabetes educator can provide feedback to the individual regarding monitoring and recording blood sugars as new skills are taught.

I believe that involving people who are diagnosed with diabetes in their own healthcare is essential from the beginning of their diagnosis. My hope is that you can see why knowledge and assertiveness in your own diabetes management is crucial, as I use my life story as an example to learn from. My life has been sweet.

Website: www.letskickdiabetes.org

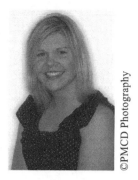
©PMCD Photography

Chapter 14   *by Jen Nash, DClinPsy*

My Journey from Feeling 'Different' to Feeling Inspired

Hi. My name's Jen and I'm a person with type 1 diabetes.

In the same way as those who have the courage to stand up in a twelve-step recovery programme, such as Alcoholics Anonymous, and say this, it has taken me about twenty years of my life since diagnosis to say this sentence without cringing or having an overwhelming sense of wanting to hide the fact that I feel I am *different*.

I was diagnosed, at age six, in London, England, where I still live today, twenty-four years later. The part I remember most clearly is the thirst: crazy, insatiable, unquenchable thirst. Getting up in the middle of the night to drink cup after cup of water from the bathroom sink, knowing this wasn't "normal," but too young to know what to do about it.

My Mum noticed changes in me, too. I'd lost weight and lacked energy and my usual "twinkle" had gone somehow. The moment of realisation occurred one morning, when I couldn't eat my breakfast cereal. I was a child who adored my food, so this seemed to be the final straw that something was really wrong. My mother took me to the family doctor, who did a urine test and said the word "diabetes" – a strange, adult word that I would hear many times over the days, weeks and years to come.

We went to the local hospital where I met Teresa, my Diabetes Specialist Nurse and Dr. Pasowicz, my Paediatric Endocrinologist, known as "Dr. P." for short. I remember the diagnosis being shared with my mum, dad, and me.

My father cried and said, "I'd do anything for her." It was the first time in my short life that I had seen him cry and to think of this memory now brings tears. I knew this "diabetes" was an adult thing, a big deal, but I was determined to face it head on – and the determination it fostered, remains with me today.

This attitude was helped by my parents, who were very encouraging of me gaining independence with caring for my diabetes, and I thank them for that. Straight away, I wanted to prove to everyone that I could "do" diabetes – quickly learning how to test my blood sugar and to inject insulin myself. I remember feeling very proud of the certificate I received the first time I completed an insulin injection independently. I attended a Children's Diabetes Day at the hospital soon after that, where I met a girl, older than I, who still needed her parent to inject her. I felt very surprised, and sorry for her. And also pleased, and quite proud, that I had mastered it. Over the years, I would often say it was lucky that I got diagnosed with diabetes and not my sister, who was very scared of needles.

Funnily enough, I don't remember much pain with the injections, although I'm sure there was some, as needles were much longer and wider on those old-fashioned syringes than the ultra-fine ones we have access to today. The "pain" of diabetes has never featured as a big deal for me. Over the years, when people found out about having to inject twice (now four times) a day, a response often was, "Ooh, doesn't it hurt?" I can understand why they would ask, but for me I think the *emotional* "hurt" of diabetes was more powerful – the feeling of being different from others.

Following the diagnosis, I was scared to return to school for a while, wanting my mum to connect with my teacher in the morning for me to feel safe. I remember crying and running into the arms of my head teacher one day when I really couldn't manage it. It's hard to think about that scared little girl, in this adult world of needles, hospitals, and doctors, trying desperately to be a "good girl," do it all right and put on a brave face. But inside, I was feeling scared and alone, and oh so *different* from the others.

The diabetes diet back then was one to "feed" the twice-daily insulin regimen, not the other way round, as it is now with four or more injections or with an insulin pump. It was rather like a diet sheet – with "exchanges" – a food with ten grams of carbohydrate was one exchange. I think I had an allowance of about ten exchanges a day. I had to eat a certain amount of carbohydrate exchanges at each meal and at regular snack times, whether I was hungry or not. Whilst, at the time I don't remember minding too much, I think this interfered with my ability to listen to my body's natural signals for hunger, which was to cause problems with my eating as I grew older.

The need to eat regularly meant I would have to eat "biscuits" (something like American shortbread cookies) at school at random times during the day.

My teachers were always very supportive and encouraging, and my mum would buy me a lovely new biscuit tin for my classroom every school year. But none of these could stop the feeling of being different, feeling all my classmates' eyes on my back as I walked to the front of the class to get my snack. I felt both fortunate (I knew my friends were very envious at how "lucky" I was that I could eat in class!) and also acutely *different*, as these were the moments that I felt the odd one out.

I found the transition to high school quite difficult. I wasn't in a class with friends from my previous school and was excluded, a little, from my old familiar friendship groups. Again, I felt alone and *different*, that I didn't fit in. I had started to travel to and from school on my own and I liked the freedom of this, and began to buy myself all the sweet foods I didn't have access to at home. There was a sweet shop about fifteen minutes from my home, and I would buy two or three chocolate bars at a time and eat them on the way home. Sometimes, if my Mum was out when I got home, I would make hot buttered toast. I think eating these foods made me feel less alone. Food was my "friend," a way of comforting myself during those difficult days of not fitting in.

In my teens and early twenties, I had lots of ups and downs with my diabetes. At times, when I really valued how important it was, I would take many blood sugar tests a day, record them diligently, and even draw charts of my results. I got a lot of praise from my doctor for this, which I enjoyed. And then, at other times, whilst I never totally ignored my diabetes, I did the minimum I needed to. I just wanted to pretend that I wasn't different; that I was "normal" just like everyone else.

My transition from the Children's to the Adults Service at hospital was a tricky one. I was growing up and didn't feel particularly able to discuss my frustrations with diabetes with my health care team. I knew they were committed and dedicated and I knew they were doing their best, but sometimes I felt like I just went there to be "checked up on." I felt distant and quite alone with it all.

I went to university and pretty much stopped going to my diabetes appointments. I think I'd lost faith and rebelled a bit. I was away from home and thought, *I'm fine, I'll think about diabetes another day.* The years at university were interesting ones, with the highs and lows that are an inevitable part of being away from home, and finding your own way in the world. I had decided to pursue a degree in Psychology, and then specialise in Clinical Psychology, not in any way (consciously, anyway) making a link between my diabetes and my chosen career interests. I felt I was here to "help" people in some way, and knew that I was interested in figuring myself out, as well as helping others figure themselves out, so psychology seemed like the obvious choice.

My clinical psychology training was very demanding, both personally and professionally. I found the subject matter inspiring and learned much about how to make links between my inner and outer world – and how my emotions and thoughts are important and need to be taken notice of, to ensure that I choose actions and behaviours that support me. This helped a great deal with my relationship with diabetes. I learned a lot about myself and how to apply these ideas in my own life, and began seeing (and still continue to see) a therapist who helps me on this journey.

When I qualified, I decided that I wanted to work with people with diabetes. I knew from my training that I liked working individually with clients and seeing them gain relief from their problems. But I also found I got restless going to the same National Health Service hospital department or clinic five days a week. I liked the idea of doing lots of different things with my working week – writing, educating and inspiring – as well as working therapeutically with clients. Based in London, I also liked the idea of not having to commute into town by public transport every day!

So I set up a service called "Positive Diabetes" with the mission to "Provide those living with diabetes with the knowledge and information they need to bring about positive improvements to their emotional life." This venture began simply as a Website, and I began writing articles for other diabetes information sites and forums and speaking at diabetes charity events, whilst developing my own range of self-help guides. The idea was to give people with diabetes permission to acknowledge that life with diabetes can be tough. As I was both a patient and a professional, this message really seemed to connect with people and I quickly built up a large following, with people finding me from all over the world.

In two short years I have grown my service into a thriving practice, and I do a whole range of different activities now, that continually excite and inspire me. These include speaking for diabetes charities, teaching and training of healthcare professionals, writing expert columns for diabetes information Websites, writing self-help programmes for sites such as www.DiabetesDaily.com and selling my own online self-help products and programmes. I've developed my own "Positive Diabetes Home Study System" (which can be found on my Website – listed at the end of this chapter) which I developed in response to people who wanted to work with me but who weren't based in the United Kingdom. It allows people to have a taste of what working with a psychologist is like, without having to take the scary step of walking into a therapist's office. (I've been there myself and know that feeling well!)

This journey has been an exciting and creative process, with a huge number of highs and lows – but I find it immensely rewarding to be able to help people and work in a way that suits me, whilst also getting paid for it. I am currently writing a book about the emotional impact of diabetes, which is due to be published by Wiley-Blackwell Publishers in 2012. I always thought I would love to write a book, but only if I had something interesting to say! Well, it looks as if diabetes has given me that.

So, what about the future? I've recently turned thirty and I have much optimism for the years ahead in my life with diabetes. I am hopeful that a cure will be found and that I will be in a position to take advantage of that.

When I was growing up I used to think, *Diabetes will never stop me from doing anything I want to do.* And, actually, it really hasn't. I went travelling at nineteen years old to Australia with my sister. I've been to university twice and gained a doctoral degree. I feel privileged to have found love. I've completed a half-marathon and a sprint triathlon (which feels even better, as I was never particularly sporty growing up!). I've been a Finalist in the MIND – Mental Health Charity Journalism Awards – for my writing on the topic of reducing the stigma associated with mental health problems.

I feel proud of my achievements, and can see that, in some ways, I used to think of diabetes as the enemy; now, I think of it as a relationship. Like any relationship, it needs time and attention to be a healthy one. Some days you are seemingly doing everything "right" but somehow the magic isn't there. But by giving it time, noticing patterns, doing more of what works and less of what doesn't – it is possible to reach a healthy balance. Okay, so my A1C isn't "perfect." My diet needs work some days, and often there are times when I know I need to exercise, but I just can't be bothered. But over the years I've come to a peace about that. I don't believe perfection exists.

The journey of diabetes has been full of highs and lows and, no doubt, will continue to be so. My work as a Clinical Psychologist has taught me that everyone has something to contend with – if it's not a health problem, it's a self-doubt . . . or a regret . . . or a misfortune . . . or an insecurity.

We are all on our own path in this life and I'm not ashamed that diabetes has been a part of mine. Diabetes has made me incredibly determined; that sense of being *different* that it fostered, has actually enabled me to have the courage to step out of the norm and create something that is benefiting others with diabetes all over the world. I think that's pretty sweet!

Website: www.PositiveDiabetes.com

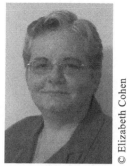

© Elizabeth Cohen

Chapter 15 *by Vanessa Nemeth, MS, MA*

Daily Choices, Daily Challenges

My Diabetes Story

I am a fifty-seven-year-old woman and have been living with type 2 diabetes since my late twenties. I work as an information systems engineer and live in New England with my spouse of seventeen years and three wonderful dogs.

Diabetes has always been "part of the family," and often feels like an additional family member. It has demands and needs like a person. I have to think about it, plan around it, and fit it into work, home life, and fun with family and friends. I need to make sure I have my medications and food with me at lunch meetings at work, on a long commute or trapped in traffic, and I often schedule my social events around when the meal is being served and what is being served. A particular challenge is travelling and vacations, when I also have to pack for it.

Diabetes has also been part of my family history. My father had the disease and his mom died of diabetes complications before I was born. Although no one in my mom's immediate family had diabetes, her aunt's husband was very sick with the disease. As a teenager, I saw him become wheelchair bound and eventually lose his legs, then his life, to diabetes. Diabetes became a scary word for me.

Then, it was my turn. I was diagnosed with diabetes shortly after my twenty-ninth birthday. I had just had my yearly physical. The careful voice on the answering machine asked that I please call back, because the doctor

155

needed to talk to me, as some test results were out of range. The initial call was followed by more lab tests and then the diagnosis I was dreading to hear: "You have diabetes."

I should not have been surprised. For several years I had been struggling with weight gain, sluggishness, excessive thirst, mood swings, and getting up many times during the night to use the bathroom. I also had been diagnosed with *hypothyroidism* and had problems with my menstrual cycle.

At first I thought, *Okay, all I need to do is take a pill. How bad can that be? At least I don't have to take insulin shots . . . I'm not that fat; it shouldn't matter.* I struggled with the doctor's recommendations to go on an aggressive diet and exercise program. No matter what I tried, I kept putting the pounds on. My weight ballooned to 235 pounds, and at 5 feet 3 inches tall, that is a lot of weight to carry around. After a while, I felt that I had come to a dead end. I felt exhausted, frustrated, and demoralized.

Then, one evening, I got a call from friends who asked that I go to the airport and pick up a "special package." I had no idea what this package was and why it had to be picked up that same evening, but I followed instructions. When I got to the airport, I was surprised to find a little black lab, sitting in a large crate waiting for me! I was thrilled by the surprise; I had wanted a pup for some time. I named the dog "Curly" and she became my best friend and exercise companion. I played with her and took her for long walks after work. I immediately started noticing improved blood sugar readings, and my mood improved significantly. Soon after, my weight started to slowly come off!

These exercise-induced changes helped me realize that there was a lot I could do to manage my diabetes! That realization led me to seriously start educating myself about diabetes and what worked best for me in terms of diet, exercise and balancing work and family demands.

My new outlook and regimen worked well for a long time. I managed my diabetes with oral medications, exercise and diet for many years. However, as middle age approached, good management became increasingly difficult and my A1C began to creep up. I resisted the advice of my physician, for at least a year, to add a daily insulin injection in the evening, but eventually I relented.

My First Insulin Shot

I remember my first insulin shot really well. Agreeing that I needed the insulin injections required me to reach a new level of acceptance of my disease. Yes, I had diabetes, but now I also had to take insulin injections as well. It was 9:30 PM and my spouse and I were feeling uneasy and apprehensive. I had listened carefully to all the instructions I received, but doubts lingered in the back on my mind . . . *what if I didn't react like everyone else? Would I wake up in the middle of the night because something went wrong? What if I didn't wake up?* Finally, deciding that I trusted my doctor and realizing I had tried everything else possible to manage my diabetes, I chose a spot on my stomach, took a deep breath, and gave myself the shot.

That was about eight years ago. I have been taking insulin shots with every meal since then and injecting has become routine. I am glad I took a positive approach to my self-management and realized that these injections were my path to better control and fewer complications from this disease. Knowing I am doing the best I can to treat this disease also liberates me from some of the stress and worry about the future. There's nothing to feel guilty about – I'm on it!

With each challenge, I try to keep the end goal – staying well with diabetes – in mind. A serious challenge was keeping my shots straight. This required a lot of focus and mindfulness! I once had the awful experience of confusing my short- and long-acting insulins, and I overdosed on short-acting insulin. Luckily, I noticed the error as soon as I put the syringe down. I immediately called my diabetes care emergency line and they were able to instruct me on what to do to avoid having severe *hypoglycemia*. That incident was very scary, and I learned a lot from it. I started marking my insulin pens and made a habit of reading the label and saying out loud which insulin I was about to inject.

An additional challenge with the insulin injections was keeping my weight under control. After eight years of injecting, my doctor recommended I consider an aggressive diabetes management program offered by the Joslin Diabetes Center in Boston, Massachusetts.

Fine-tuning

The new program consisted of weekly classes at the clinic. First, a one-hour session at the gym, where we learned how to maximize the effectiveness of exercise by combining aerobic and strength training exercises. The gym session was followed by a lecture/discussion, where we covered different topics ranging from proper nutrition to emotional well-being. These well-rounded classes also included an evaluation and adjustments of our medication protocols.

No two people in our class of fifteen members took the same combinations of medications. My protocol adjustments resulted in me injecting three different medications, for a total of up to nine injections a day! At first I was intimidated by this regimen. Did I have enough body surface to administer all these shots? I resented the daily preparation of medications that I needed to take to work, or anywhere I went. I almost felt sorry for myself. The bruises from all the injections were hard to look at . . . but I stuck with it. The support within our group, and from my spouse, was outstanding. I was not doing this alone.

157

Every week, for three months, I made the long trip to the clinic. Each session started with a weigh-in, and almost every week I had lost weight! At the end of the program, I was the thinnest I had ever been as an adult. My A1C, cardiovascular endurance and percentage of body fat were also tremendously improved! I felt like I had found the formula which I needed to add active years to my life.

The Insulin Pump

I was able to successfully stay on this nutrition and exercise regimen for about fourteen months. However, the demands of nine shots a day became disheartening and burdensome. I couldn't stand looking at myself in the mirror because of the bruising.

I mentioned these concerns to my physician, and we discussed the pros and cons of switching to an insulin pump. My physician thought I was a good candidate for the device. I had managed to keep a very rigorous regimen with all the injections and she thought I would be able to manage the requirements of being on the pump as well. It seemed like a good option to consider because it would eliminate the need for nine daily injections.

I immediately signed up for a pump training program and within several weeks I had received the pump and educational material. I was ready to do the switch! The trickiest part of the switch from injections to the pump was figuring out the various metabolic rates. This required fasting, which I did over several weekends, so it wouldn't affect my driving or ability to concentrate at work. After my metabolic rates were established, and the pump was properly fine-tuned, I was happy to find that my body responded very well to my new regimen.

After four months on the pump (which I sometimes refer to of as my "new and improved pancreas"), I am using a fraction of the insulin I used previously and my A1C is the lowest it has been in a decade! The only drawback is what I call the "pump tax." I gained four pounds within a week of the switch and I have not been able to take them off yet. Even though I've gained some weight (which I'll need to lose again), the freedom, benefits, and well-being of using the pump are priceless.

The model I use is submersible. I can get into the pool or go to the beach without worrying. I enjoy not having to go through the hassle of packing injections, pen needles and the rest of the paraphernalia every time I leave the house. No more getting to work after an hour commute and having to turn around because I forgot my insulin kit. I love not being bruised any longer.

I've been asked if the pump isn't a constant reminder of diabetes and being "sick." For me, diabetes is a condition I manage – and yes, it is a progressive condition – but I have an incredible ability to influence a lot of the outcomes. Keeping tight management of my blood sugar is the best thing I can do to improve my outcomes. Being on the pump helps me achieve that goal. So, for me, the pump is a constant reminder that I am doing the most I can to *keep myself as healthy as can be* with diabetes.

Exercise and Its Challenges

The other piece of my successful diabetes management program is exercise. I've never been the trim gal in a pretty spandex outfit jogging down the street with my iPod tunes setting my stride. I am not a fan of the gym either, but I've come to love exercise! It makes me feel good physically and mentally. I've come to expect and enjoy the reward of good blood sugar readings.

However, I have struggled with exercise-related injuries through the years. I've dealt with inflammation and tendinitis in my heels and elbows, a torn meniscus and herniated lower back discs. All these injuries presented challenges to weight management and blood sugar control, not to mention battling a tendency toward the "Why me?" syndrome. I've learned that injuries are going to happen, so, I've tried to figure out what are the safest and most enjoyable types of exercise for me. When I've been seriously injured, I resorted to water jogging at the local YMCA. The water jogging gave me a good aerobic workout and it helped me emotionally, knowing that I was still being relatively active, despite the injuries and difficulties outside the pool.

Once I was on my path to recovery, I used the pool to start working on strength training exercises, provided by my physical therapist. Fortunately, I have enough space in my home for an elliptical strider, an exercise bike and an assortment of hand weights and resistance bands. I've learned to do strength training through various classes, and instructional media. I fight the monotony by using videos or DVDs shot outdoors, providing the feeling that I am biking down the California coast or struggling up a mountainside in Hawaii. Other times, I play tapes of my favorite dance music, assembled through the years. I also switch up my routine in the summertime, when I favor long walks outdoors over staying in my home gym.

Another component of my exercise routine is my lunch-time walk at work. I take a thirty-minute walking break almost every day – religiously! Even if I don't get to my after-work routine, at least I have a thirty minute walk under my belt, which also improves my work stress levels.

I've come to understand that I need to exercise because it is critical for good diabetes management and cardiovascular health. I've learned to fight the "negatives" – feeling sorry for myself or becoming frustrated when I get injured or feeling resentful about time demands. It is hard to go to work, endure a long commute, take time to exercise, cook a healthy meal, and deal with family demands every day . . . but that is what it takes. Being positive allows me to come up with creative ways to accomplish this.

Nutrition and Weight Challenges

When it comes to dieting or weight loss, what haven't I tried? I've tried Atkins™ to Richard Simmons, Weight Watchers®, Jenny Craig®, nutritionist programs, vegetarianism, and many other approaches; I even tried a women's weight support group. They kicked me out of the group when I hit 199 pounds because they thought I was too thin!

All these programs taught me something and helped in some way. Over the years, I have wheedled my weight down from the 230s in my late twenties and early thirties, to the 190s in my forties and now in the 170s in my late fifties. I do have a goal to get down to the 150s within the next year. The formula that has worked the best for me is planning my meals and tracking what I eat and my exercise. I will lose weight if I keep my daily intake to 1200-1300 calories a day *and* I exercise *vigorously* a minimum of five days a week. Through the program at the Joslin Diabetes Center, I've learned to put meals together that fall in this caloric range. I scan Websites or the Sunday paper for recipes that I can use or adjust. I try to avoid monotony by switching things around, and not preparing the same meals week after week. I like having a repertoire of at least two dozen dinner time meals which I can choose from that I know my spouse will enjoy, too. This, in turn, helps me figure out what I need to shop for. I also like making large batches on weekends so I can keep frozen "extras." I know I can easily defrost a good meal, if I am thrown a curve ball and the day does not turn out as planned!

Meal planning is one aspect of my nutrition program and the other is tracking my calories; that is the best tool I've found for weight loss. There it is – just me and my diary. I know exactly what I've eaten and when I ate it. For a while, I also spent some time tracking how I was feeling and found some interesting patterns.

For example, I discovered that stepping into the house after a long commute in the evening was a danger time for me. Now that I know that, I incorporate an afternoon snack into my diet that takes care of the urge to stand in front of the refrigerator or pantry and start nibbling, out of control, the minute I get home. Another pattern for me was overeating at parties or when going out. I've learned that if I have a small snack before I leave the house, then I am not starving, and I have an easier time keeping myself in control. I've learned these things from keeping a record and tracking what I eat. I feel that anyone can do this. If you are totally honest, then you can see the challenges and figure out how to fix it!

I also found online tools helpful and there are many to choose from. I've found SparkPeople.com very helpful and it's free! Besides allowing users to track foods, the site offers exercise advice and has a terrific online community. One can join an on-going discussion or blog about your situation or join a fitness challenge. It is motivating to talk to others or read about others who are struggling with similar issues.

While I don't track what I eat all the time, I always go back to it when I start going off course. For that reason, I weigh myself at least three times a week. Weight has a sneaky way of creeping back on. I find it easier to deal with it when it is just one or two pounds and not ten! When I start going off track, I will log my food intake for a while – typically until I reach my target weight.

I have no "secret weapon" to successful diabetes management. I just follow a consistent, pro-active regimen. As part of this regimen, I see the diabetes doctor or nurse practitioner every three months. I go for a dilated eye exam every year, and I check in with my nutritionist on a regular basis. With their help and encouragement, I have learned, through trial and error, what works best for me. I have also learned to change things up and "keep it fresh." This applies to my meals and my exercise program as well. I have learned that I need to juggle nutrition and exercise every day, that I need to take care of these things at work and at home, and when I am busy and when I am not. There isn't a day off.

Dealing with diabetes is not a "life sentence," or something to suffer with for a lifetime. I accept the fact that I have a medical condition and that I have the ability to make good choices. I have had times when the challenges felt like too much, but I try to stay positive and look for "work-arounds." There is always another way to *work around* the problem.

I have realized over the years that the way I approach the challenges has a lot to do with my success. I am motivated to choose to exercise and continue to manage my weight by knowing I am doing all I can to stay healthy and because I feel better! After twenty-eight years with the disease, my diabetes is currently under the best management I've ever had, and I feel pretty lucky to have kept the major complications at bay. This is what drives me – the thought that my daily choices yield better outcomes over my daily challenges. I can't control the future, but for now, I am enjoying the health I have!

I just read in the local paper that there is a new Pilates class starting up at the Y this Fall. Maybe I'll sign up . . .

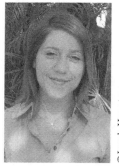

©Jacob Hauptman

Chapter 16   *by Alexis Pollack*

From Diabetes Rock Bottom to Running on Insulin

It's 6:00 AM on a May morning in San Diego, and I'm standing on a platform above hundreds of eager cyclists at the San Diego Tour de Cure. The annual bike ride is the American Diabetes Association's fundraiser for diabetes research. The folks below me listen as I review safety information for their upcoming 100-mile journey. I look out to the crowd and spot dozens of cyclists wearing what's called a "Red Rider" jersey - a bright red bike jersey that proudly displays "I Ride with Diabetes" on the back. Each person with diabetes who rides in the Tour gets one for free. I'm wearing mine, too, having had type 1 diabetes for almost twenty years. I ask the crowd to give a cheer for those riding with diabetes today, and the people below erupt in support.

I serve as the volunteer chair of the Tour de Cure, and had devoted hundreds of hours of volunteer work to make it successful. As I look around the colorful starting line, I see the logo for my company (a diabetes pharmaceutical manufacturer) on several of the banners at the event. I also see many faces in the crowd that I've met through my hobby, a diabetes blog called *I Run on Insulin* that has connected me with hundreds of other people with diabetes in the online community.

Beyond the smiles and bikes though, I see the wonderful life I have built for myself around diabetes. I see my successful career, my community leadership, my passion for advocacy and education, and my friends and family, all brought together by diabetes. I see my health and my ability to live well with type 1 diabetes, and the fact that I have turned my diagnosis into a blessing. My rich and fulfilling life has been shaped around having type 1 diabetes, so much so that it has become my work, my philanthropy, and my hobby. Though I'm happy and healthy now, my life wasn't always this way.

Ten years ago, I was very ill and in a hospital bed. I had an IV in each arm, one with an insulin drip, the other with rehydrating fluids. My step-mom lay sleeping near me on a hospital cot, too afraid for my life to leave my side. The night before, I had nearly died from *diabetic ketoacidosis* (DKA), a dangerous condition in which chronic high blood sugar causes an acid build-up in the bloodstream that can be fatal. I hadn't checked my blood sugar in weeks and only taken my insulin sporadically. This would turn out to be my "diabetes rock bottom," but it would also be the moment I turned my life around. The moment I chose to live well with diabetes and let it inspire me to live the fulfilling life I had always dreamed about.

How did I get from that hospital bed to the podium at Tour? It was a journey, and it is my diabetes story which continues on to this day. And it all started with a trip to the Mayo Clinic in Rochester, Minnesota, when I was just ten years old.

I grew up in a sunny San Diego neighborhood. Like many Southern California kids, I didn't know how lucky I was until long after I'd grown up. While other kids spent summers at traditional camps, my sisters and I were at surf camp, learning how to "hang ten" in the Pacific Ocean. I am the middle of three sisters, and all of us were active tomboys growing up. I can remember hours playing outside our house on our bikes and rollerblades. My sisters and I would often craft elaborate fairy tales in which we all fought over who would play the Knight in Shining Armor. There was nary a doll to be found in our house – my sisters and I preferred to spend hours on end tearing up the beach and basketball court. Looking back, I can't believe how good we had it.

Things changed for my family, though, in 1992, when I was nine years old. My parents separated and what followed were years of a painful divorce process. Suddenly, our lives were split into visitation rights, moving houses, and teasing from kids at school about our new arrangement. Our home life, once so idyllic, was turned completely upside down.

It was that same year I distinctly remember knowing something was wrong with me. Every time my sisters and I would come in from playing outside, I would guzzle a pitcher of water and still be dying of thirst. When our family would sit down for a Saturday night movie, I'd have to use the bathroom at least five times before the film's end. One awful day after karate practice, I remember not making it to the bathroom at my dad's apartment. My dad dunked me and my soggy pants in the bathtub and I remember sobbing hysterically. I cried, not just because I was embarrassed, but because my dad felt so badly.

He thought it was his fault that he hadn't asked if I needed to use the restroom before leaving practice that night. In reality, he had no idea that I'd been trying to hide my excessive thirst and urination for weeks at that point. Even at the age of nine, I just knew something wasn't right. Later that year, my fears would be confirmed with a diagnosis of type 1 diabetes.

Every year, my mother would take my sisters and me to spend Christmas with our grandparents in Rochester, Minnesota, home of the world-famous Mayo Clinic. In what only can be described as a truly bizarre twist of irony, my retired grandfather had spent his career at the Mayo Clinic as a top endocrinologist. When we arrived in Rochester to spend the Christmas of 1992 with them, my symptoms were full-blown and I could no longer hide them. My mom noticed how often I had to come inside from sledding to use the restroom and the pitchers of water I downed at every meal. My mom knew something was wrong and my grandfather, with his years of experience, suspected type 1 diabetes.

The day I was diagnosed plays back in my mind like an old home video. I'm dressed in my favorite Christmas sweater (the one with the gingerbread house on it, ironic now that I think back on it). My mom, grandpa, and I went to the Mayo Clinic, although I thought I'm just getting a routine check-up at the special Minnesota hospital. The nurse jabbed my finger with a lancet and I pulled my hand back, yelping in pain. She guided my finger to the test strip, which, unbeknownst to, me is the first of thousands of strips I would see in my lifetime.

Although I don't remember the exact number that came back on the glucose meter, I do remember it was in the 200+ mg/dL range. My grandfather stood, looking down at the meter, his hands in his pockets, nervously shifting his weight from side to side as he waited for the number to appear. When it did, he showed no emotion, just flatly read the number out loud. My grandpa and mom left to go speak with a doctor.

When they came back, a nurse accompanied them, toting a very big needle. They needed to draw blood from my arm, my mom said, and that's when my ten-year-old self lost it. Screaming and crying, I nearly had to be pinned down while the needle was jabbed in to my arm to draw a blood test that would conclusively seal my diagnosis.

My mom and grandfather disappeared again, this time for a very long time. I remember that the nurse had put on a Disney cartoon to keep me entertained while they went to speak with the doctor. I also remember thinking something was very, very wrong when the movie ended and the nurse had to put on another one. We went home that night, burdened with the arsenal of new diabetes supplies, and it was the first time no one in my house had a cookie for dessert.

165

Our Christmas vacation was extended several extra weeks at my grandpa's house, where, under his expert care, we learned how to manage my diabetes. My mom quickly learned how to mix my Regular and NPH insulins, how to adjust them for my blood sugars, and that cake, candy, and cookies were now off limits for the middle daughter.

We returned home to San Diego, where I was lucky enough to be attending a private elementary school with a nurse who could administer my insulin and perform glucose checks. My father was a surgeon and, although his field was unrelated to diabetes, he was certainly well-versed in managing patients. Right away, I became his patient at home. My dad would encourage me to manage my diabetes on my own, so that I would have the freedom to be more like a normal kid.

In fact, it was at my dad's house that I remember doing my first injection on my own. Perched on his giant desk chair, I warily eyed the orange-capped syringe. I was about twelve years old at the time, just two years into living with diabetes. I wanted to be allowed to go to sleepovers, like other girls my age did, but because I couldn't inject on my own, I was only allowed to stay over at one friend's house whose mom was a nurse. If I could do my own injections though, I'd be allowed at the other sleepovers and who knows where else! Doing my own shots was going to mean independence. So that day, at my father's desk (which perhaps was providing some grown-up inspiration), I pulled off the orange cap, pinched up my skin on my stomach, and jammed the needle in. *Freedom*, I thought. *Now I'm in control of this thing. I do my own blood sugar tests, my own shots, and now I can go anywhere and do anything.*

Looking back, those first few years with diabetes weren't so bad (although I am sure my parents would disagree, since they carried the biggest burden of worry). I had my grandpa to call when we had questions, my dad's medical knowledge at all times, a private school with access to a nurse, and good insurance that paid for my supplies. I recall having good hemoglobin A1Cs for those early years, and a tremendous amount of support from my school, friends, and family. However, things would change as I cntered high school, and the bottom fell out of my world.

It was the summer of 1996, and my dad pulled us three girls and his girlfriend, who would soon be his wife, into the living room. He told us that the cancer he'd beaten a few years before had returned, but that he was aggressively seeking treatment and that he was going to be okay. It was right before we left for a family vacation, and I remember him looking happy and healthy. Just one year after that, though, my father would become a gaunt shadow of that man, fighting a losing battle to the cancer that would eventually consume him.

In December of 1997, just two months after my dad and my step-mom married, my father succumbed to his illness. I was fifteen years old and in the middle of my freshman year of high school. As I grappled with the earth-shattering change in my life, my diabetes management was the furthest thing from my mind. It would stay that way until I almost lost my own life to DKA.

I returned to my freshman year of high school confused, scared, and devastated by the loss of my father. My older sister had returned to college, so I was living at home with my mom and younger sister. Like many kids who experience loss at a young age, I was truly incapable of processing my feelings toward my dad dying, and I acted out in a variety of ways. I broke curfew, talked back, and sulked for days on end; I certainly wasn't the most pleasant child to be around for those first years after my dad was gone. And diabetes? It couldn't have been further from my mind. I would skip my glucose checks at school. I'd conveniently leave my insulin in my locker at lunchtime. No one else had to deal with this stupid disease, so why should I?

It was around that time that I also discovered a very dangerous thing about diabetes: you can have elevated blood sugars for a long time without any immediate serious consequences. Sure, I often felt tired and thirsty, but it wasn't like refusing to test my blood sugar at lunch caused me to fall over dead. I thought I could get away without checking for days at a time, taking sporadic doses of insulin that must have just barely kept me going. This dangerous viewpoint about my diabetes management is a trap that many people fall into. Not taking care of your diabetes today doesn't always mean there is an immediate punishment, but over time, uncontrolled diabetes is silently ravaging your body.

Diabetes requires that we think in the long-term, but to a teenage girl, angry at the world for taking her father and for having this dumb disease, tomorrow didn't matter. I cared that right now I didn't feel like testing my blood sugar and it just wasn't going to happen.

Although I was lying to myself and my family and friends about how bad my control was, my A1Cs told the true story. By age sixteen, my A1C was routinely coming back at 13 percent and 14 percent, meaning my average blood sugars were nearly 400 mg/dL all the time. I was a ticking time bomb, and in retrospect, I'm surprised that it took so long for me to hit DKA, given the length of time I was in such poor control.

It was the summer of 2001, and I had gone out to a party with friends the night before. Like many teenagers, we were just beginning to experiment with alcohol. I remember I'd indulged in some sickly sweet cocktail of orange juice and vodka, and had awakened the next morning violently ill. No matter what I did, I couldn't stop vomiting. My head was spinning and I knew this wasn't just a bad night of drinking – something was truly wrong.

My older sister was home from college, and her boyfriend, who would later become my brother-in-law, was visiting for the first time. I called for my older sister to bring me my glucose meter, which practically had to be dusted off because I hadn't used it in so long. I tested my blood, and the meter read over 500 mg/dL. I took a random shot of insulin, but I knew I was past being able to care for myself.

With my sister's insistence, we called my step-mom to take me to the hospital, as my mother was out of town; ironically, in Minnesota visiting my grandparents. I was so weak, my sister and brother-in-law had to practically carry me to the car, bolstering me upright on either side as I hobbled. My step-mom sped to the hospital, or at least tried to. She was so distraught at my condition and I was so out of sorts that we got lost, right there in our hometown, on the way to the emergency department. We both look back on that scary day and laugh at how long it took us to get to the hospital.

I was admitted to the emergency ward and treated for diabetic ketoacidosis right away. My chronic high blood sugars had finally caught up with me, and my body was shutting down. I remember a fitful, painful night in the ER with what seemed liked dozens of pokes – finger sticks, blood draws, and IVs going in. It was an awful experience. When I finally stabilized, weak, dehydrated, and exhausted, I was moved to a hospital room on the main floor while I recovered.

I lay in that bed, IVs in both arms, feeling like an utter and complete failure. Diabetes had beaten me. I had let it creep up on me and almost take my life. I had ignored it and pushed it away until it revolted and forced me to pay attention. This was my diabetes rock bottom; I had to hit it, so that I could battle my way back to health.

Those days in the hospital gave me a lot of time to think. Worried friends floated in and out, bringing flowers and cards. They looked at me just as they should have: as a sick person not in control of her health. I hated knowing they thought of me as "the sick kid," the girl with diabetes who will always be held back by this disease.

Years later, someone would ask me what my diabetes "a-ha" moment was: when was the moment when I realized I had to change? Although I will always look back at the time in the hospital as my "a-ha" moment, it's important to know that it was the actions I took after leaving the hospital that changed my life. It was the journey of education, understanding, and empowerment that I embarked on that would truly change my diabetes management and my life. Those awful days in the hospital, feeling like I had let everyone down, including myself, were the catalyst I needed to change my dire trajectory.

After spending five days in the hospital recovering from DKA, I was released in July of 2001. I had graduated from high school just a month earlier, and was headed to college in Los Angeles in just two short months. My entire life was about to change, as I left my childhood home and headed to college, but it would be my diabetes management that would undergo the most drastic transformation.

Immediately after my release from the hospital, I began more aggressive self monitoring. I dusted off that rarely-used glucose meter and began testing. I realized that, without the information of where my blood sugar was, I couldn't make any intelligent decisions. At that time in my life, I only saw two types of numbers on the meter: bad and good (also known as "High/Low" or "Normal Range"). Basic as it may seem, the simple act of testing was more attention to my diabetes than I'd given it in years.

My family sought out the best endocrinologist in town to help me improve my health. I soon found myself in the office of a doctor whose demeanor carried both deep compassion and understanding for his patients, as well as the authoritative stature of a parent bent on teaching a wayward kid a thing or two about discipline. This was the first physician I had ever seen who gave equal parts kindness and tough love. He took the time to explain to me where I was headed on my current path of ignoring my diabetes, and also appropriately enticed me with the promise that good control meant I could do anything I wanted: go to college, travel the world, have a boyfriend, and have a successful career.

It was this doctor, and his staff who began to teach me that controlling my diabetes, not denying it, is what would truly set me free. After years of doctors uselessly shoving scary statistics down my throat, the compassion of this doctor, and his staff, helped me realize that taking care of my diabetes was honoring and valuing myself. They also understood that diabetes was hard to live with. They never expected perfection from me, just effort and a willingness to learn and accept.

Looking back at the changes I made to my life in order to take care of my diabetes, becoming a patient at this office was one of key factors of my success. It taught me that having the right healthcare provider can be as important as taking your medications. I found that my healthcare team had to be part of my network of support, and also a guiding light in my journey with diabetes.

I went off to college in the fall of 2001 and, like many eighteen-year-olds who head to a university after so long under their parent's roof, I voraciously took in my new-found freedom. No curfew? Wow! No chores? All right! Leaving for college was, in a way, an escape from my old life. I had left the town where my father had passed away, full of painful memories, and exchanged it for a second chance on a sprawling Los Angeles campus. I had also left behind my old "diabetes self." I had been at my worst, and with the blessing of the second chance I was granted, I was determined to change my life and my health.

169

Looking back, I now realize that fresh start at college could not have come at a better time for my diabetes. I needed new surroundings, a new outlook, and a new beginning.

New friends came with college, and I made one very important choice with this new group. Everyone I met would learn up front, right away, that I had diabetes. No more hiding, no more apologizing. My introduction became "my name is Alexis, I'm from San Diego, and I have type 1 diabetes". From there, I could field questions about insulin and blood sugar and get it out of the way, up front.

Letting people know I had diabetes right away was not something my old self would have done. My old self would have been embarrassed and ashamed, worried about what people might think. But the new Alexis would no longer apologize for having this disease. This was the first step I took to letting diabetes be part of who I am. Later, it would shape the direction of my life and my success.

For many people, college is a chance to break free from the chains of high school and discover who they are, and for me, it was no different. In particular, though, I discovered a tremendous amount about my diabetes. While I was changing my major and trying various intramural sports to see what was perfect for me, I was also discovering what worked for my diabetes management. I was learning how to incorporate diabetes into my lifestyle, so that I wasn't held back by it.

I started working out in the school gym after my freshman roommate introduced me to the cardio machines. By senior year, I was running all ten sets of the stadium stairs and that was just my warm up. As I learned about exercise, I also learned about proper nutrition. I began to understand how carbohydrates and exercise affected my glucose, and how I felt after an active day with healthy eating. I was checking my blood sugar up to ten times a day, and maintaining an A1C below 7 percent. I had joined a competitive karate team, earning belts and medals aplenty.

In my four years at college, I can't believe how far I came from that sick kid in the hospital bed. I had shed fifteen pounds, worked out five days a week, and was finally in good control of my diabetes. Most importantly, I realized that, when I took control of my disease, I would be allowed to do anything I wanted, just like my doctor had promised.

One of my fondest memories of college was also an important experience in reinforcing that I could do anything I wanted with diabetes: my semester studying abroad in Spain. I'll never forget packing for that trip! I was on multiple daily injections at the time, and was told it would be easier to pack everything I needed for the five months abroad rather than trying to buy my supplies in Spain. I loaded 500 syringes into my giant suitcase, along with all my other diabetes paraphernalia needed for the long trip.

As expected, I was pulled aside right away by Spanish customs. Fortunately, I had obtained a doctor's note in Spanish, and brought backups for all my prescriptions in case my supplies were detained. Much to my relief, I was eventually let through customs, my supplies still safely with me.

I then proceeded on one of the most grand adventures of my life. The five months I spent in Spain were among the most carefree I'll ever experience. Every night, we dined and danced through the Spanish neighborhoods; every weekend, we took a train to explore another corner of Europe. Most importantly, I showed myself that I could travel the world, live with strangers, taste sangria, take midnight trains to Barcelona, and have the time of my life, even though I had diabetes. It was an experience that proved to me that diabetes didn't have to hold me back.

After graduating from college, I knew I wanted a career where I could make a difference in the world of diabetes. Diabetes is a tremendously demanding disease. We count carbohydrates, we titrate our insulin, we check our glucose, and we're constantly running through our management in our heads, trying to anticipate the next move diabetes will make. Diabetes already consumed so much of my mental energy that I was sure I wanted my work to be related to this disease. But I wasn't sure how I could build a successful career around diabetes.

Then, I landed a job at an incredible company in San Diego. My company makes several first-in-class drugs for diabetes, medications that help people live longer and better with diabetes. The beauty of working for a diabetes company was twofold. First, it provided a supportive work environment for *my* diabetes. No one looked at me funny when I tested during a meeting, no one second-guessed me when I sipped a juice box during a presentation because I was heading for a low. It was okay to have diabetes at my office. Second, I felt a deep sense of satisfaction from my work each day. Even if I had spent the day buried in spreadsheets, I felt comforted knowing my contribution helped people with diabetes at the end of the day.

Looking back on my years at the company, I realized that, like my healthcare provider, my work had become part of my network of support. By choosing to work in the diabetes field, I had a rewarding career that was also conducive to my health. My company supports people living well with diabetes, and therefore I was empowered by my workplace to maintain my diabetes health. I don't think that everyone needs to work for a diabetes company to achieve this, of course; what's important is that my work enables me to take care of my diabetes. It may be the content of the work, the work-life balance that it affords, or the supportive co-workers who helped me stay on course with diabetes. Diabetes demands constant attention, and having a place where I spend forty-plus hours a week which is supportive of my good health has been essential to my diabetes control.

My passion for diabetes advocacy and education grew as I became a bona-fide adult. I found diabetes connections in my work, and I had begun to volunteer for the American Diabetes Association's local Tour de Cure. Through that event, I was able to channel my new-found love of cycling into something positive for diabetes.

Although this volunteer work was rewarding, another place captured much of my diabetes attention: the online community. Every day, I would log on to marvelous diabetes blogs where there were hundreds of people, just like me, navigating the everyday challenges with this disease. There were athletes, mothers, writers, executives, and people who reminded me oh-so-much of that very ill young woman I had been but a short time ago. I loved to hear how other people managed specific diabetes situations. The exchange of ideas and lamentations and celebrations was camaraderie unlike anything I had experienced, and I wanted to be a part of it. I wanted to add my voice to the chorus of people living well with diabetes. That's why, in February of 2009, www.irunoninsulin.com was born.

I Run on Insulin, despite the play on words, is about far more than just running. My blog boasts the tagline of "a Website about living life to the fullest with diabetes", because I truly believe that it can be done. I believe that, even with diabetes, and perhaps *because* of having diabetes, I can indeed live a rich, fulfilling, healthy life full of all the things any person with a functioning pancreas can have. I started blogging because I wanted to connect with people who felt the same way I did, so that we could share stories, tips and tricks, and most importantly, remind each other that we are not alone.

Whenever I wonder how in the heck I'm going to get through a diabetes issue, all I have to do is log on. Immediately, I am reminded that I am *not* the first person to have to deal with this, and that I will get through it. The power of the online community is truly strength in numbers. The combined experience of thousands of patient voices is worth more than any doctor's office. When someone has lived through it, you know that you can, too. That's the power of the online community – access to hundreds of stories spoken with voices of empathy, understanding, and inspiration.

Since starting my blog in 2009, it has grown to hundreds of readers a day and led to a variety of connections and projects in the diabetes world. My blog focuses on the daily issues of living with type 1 diabetes, with special attention to sports and diabetes management. Writing my blog helps me learn more about myself and my diabetes every single day, and my readers' comments help me understand this disease more deeply with each post. When I decided to go on an insulin pump a few years ago, it was my blog and other sites that I turned to for product reviews from the patients themselves. When I ran my first half marathon in 2009, I turned to my readers for advice. Once again, I came to realize that my blog, like my job, my healthcare provider, and my volunteer work with the ADA, is yet another pillar of support for my diabetes health.

The past ten years, since my episode of DKA, have actually been a construction project. I've cobbled together a lifestyle for myself that allows me to live well with diabetes. Or perhaps, it is my diabetes that has allowed me to live well. Period.

Upon my diagnosis at age ten, I would never have said that diabetes was a blessing in disguise. Eight year later, as I lay in that hospital bed recovering from DKA, I still found it hard to accept the good in this disease. Now, as I look around at the rich life diabetes has given me, I can hardly believe all the blessings I have *because* of this disease. I have a fulfilling career, I have a passionate hobby, and I have my health. This is not to say that I don't have fears and concerns about diabetes, because I do. I worry about complications from this disease down the road. I worry about having children one day, for fear I might pass diabetes to them. I even still occasionally worry that maybe having diabetes will hold me back from something I really want to do. Those are the days when I log on to the blogs and see how other people have tackled these fears. It is truly a comfort to know all that support is just a few clicks away.

If I could go back in time to my former self, who at age eighteen found herself weak, defeated, and lonely in that hospital bed, I would tell her that she is not alone. I would tell her that she can live well with this disease. She can do anything she wants to do, but that ignoring diabetes is to ignore herself, and what is a part of who she is. I would tell her that it's not her fault, and that she doesn't need to be sorry for having diabetes. I would make sure she understood that the only tragedy would be to let it hold her back.

I think back to the day of the Tour de Cure, high above the crowd on the podium, looking over a sea of athletes who have united to fight diabetes. I think about how far I have come, about how much I have learned. I think about who I used to be and who I still want to become. I think that, without diabetes, all of this goodness, this kindness, the inspiration and love that I have found because of it, wouldn't be in my life. I am astounded at how much diabetes has given me, not taken away. In fact, it has given me the power to be my very best self.

Website: www.irunoninsulin.com

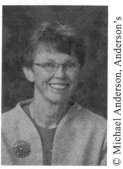

Chapter 17 *by Birgitta Rice, MS, RPh, CHES*

Walk Fast and Look Happy!

My parents, serving as Christian missionaries from Sweden to India, were spending time in Coonoor, a small, mountain resort town in southern India where there was a missionary hospital. It is very hot on the plains in India during the summer months and in anticipation of my birth, they had chosen to spend the last month of my mom's pregnancy in the mountains, where it was cooler.

One summer night, the monsoon rains and storms were just beginning over the Nilgiri Mountains in southern India. My dad was trying to bring my mother to the hospital, as I was about to be born. It was a blustery, rainy night. The strong winds were rolling in over the mountains, and trees were falling across the roads. Friends who accompanied them had to cut through trees and branches to be able to clear enough space for the Jeep to make it through on the road to the hospital, but everyone made it in one piece. And so I appeared, Inga Birgitta Olsson! As is often the case in Sweden, my middle name was the one I would be called.

My childhood was spent in India, experiencing everything from chirping crickets, snakes, and howling jackals in moonlit nights in the deep jungles of central India, to attending a Swedish boarding school with Swedish curriculum in Kodaikanal, which is located in the Nilgiri mountains in Tamil Nadu, the southernmost part of the Indian Peninsula. The Swedish school children were often invited to perform Swedish folk dances for Indian royals, or Maharajahs, visiting the sought-after resort town with a climate like that of California. I moved to Sweden, to stay, when I was twelve years old.

175

After my high school graduation, the question came – what to do next? I had decided I wanted to go into the medical field. But since I had chosen a curriculum in high school that did not include enough chemistry, math or physics, I had to study these subjects at the university over the summer and then take an entrance exam in the fall. It was a big decision to take all three subjects in one summer, but I was determined and persistent.

I took the labs and the lectures at the university in Lund. I had to find a tutor in math. My tutor lived on the fourth floor of an old, old house in Lund. There was no elevator, so every time I went there, I had to climb a small winding stairway, without landings, to get up to his apartment. I felt winded, tired and so thirsty. I often had to eat an apple on the way up to keep my mouth from completely drying up!

Diabetes was Diagnosed

It had been a very hot summer in Sweden. I noticed I was drinking a lot of water and I was hungry all the time. But I persevered and was able to finish the courses. The tests were to be given at the end of October.

My sister was a registered nurse living in Lund at the time. When I had some hours off, I would visit with her to eat my lunch and rest a bit in her apartment. Her nursing literature lined the bookshelves. I had realized that there was probably something wrong with my health, so I looked for direction in my sister's nursing books and found a few that gave me some insight. I pretty much determined it for myself that I had the symptoms of diabetes. But I wasn't ready to tell my mother.

Mother had often talked about her sister, who had had diabetes. She was twelve years old when she was diagnosed, and died from it within a fairly short time. In those days, insulin had just been discovered and patients started taking insulin injections, but they really didn't know how to monitor it. My grandfather even moved his family from northern Sweden south to Stockholm for her to be able to get the insulin injections. My mother was aware that diabetes had a hereditary component and that someone in her family might also develop diabetes.

One day, when I helped my mother with the laundry, I was so thirsty that I kept drinking water from the hose. My mother said, "Birgitta, are you *that* thirsty that you have to drink water from the hose?!"

"Yes!" I answered.

She then decided to take a sample of my urine to the pharmacy to have it tested. It came back positive for sugar in the urine. I had a feeling that she had wondered from time to time if that could be why I was so tired and not feeling well. Shortly thereafter, I saw my family physician for a check-up. He found my blood sugar to be 350 mg/dL and ordered me to enter the hospital to be treated and discharged for a life with *diabetes mellitus.*

My diabetes care, as I left the two-week-long hospital stay, was given to me by the nurse and consisted of a small 4 x 6 inch book with a list of food exchanges and a sample daily menu. Treatment was: a controlled diet, weighing and measuring all foods by grams on a letter scale and liquids with a deciliter measuring cup; one daily insulin shot in the morning; urine testing two to three times daily. To test my urine, I premeasured about a half of a teaspoon of water in a test-tube; added ten drops of urine (collected in a separate beaker); added a reagent tablet, which fizzed and bubbled for about a minute. The final color from green-yellow-orange-rust indicated the sugar concentration 0 to +3 in the urine. You can imagine that the result was seldom green because this urine was collected in the bladder during the previous three to four hours.

It was very frustrating to keep a log because of the constant sugar values. There was no way to adjust the regimen and no one to ask until the next doctor visit. Weekly, I had to sterilize the glass-syringe, the seven stainless steel needles, and the container, which was then filled with new, clean alcohol to keep the contents sterile in preparation for my daily injections.

Thank God for my mother! She was my support and strength. She helped me figure out the meal plan and how I could get the most nutrition out of the meager food plan. When I received this food plan, fifty-two years ago, there was no carbohydrate counting or distinction of fats. The diet consisted of two tablespoons of butter, two slices of bread, two starchy vegetables, two servings of protein or cheese and two glasses of milk a day. She baked, she cooked, she measured, and she helped me through the insulin reactions, which were many and hard. Now, in retrospect, I say, "No doubt, with such a meager diet!"

After finding my blood sugars very low so often, I thought maybe I didn't have diabetes anymore. Years later, that was explained to me as the "honeymoon phase" of diabetes. During this time, the pancreas may still secrete some insulin. Over time, this secretion stops and, as this happens, one requires more insulin from injections. The "honeymoon period" can last weeks or months; for me, it was a couple of months.

Then, as now, diabetes did not stop me. As I had studied violin for about seven years and played in a symphony orchestra, I kept my commitment and performed in concert on my violin (Malmö Civic Symphony Orchestra) the weekend following my initial two-week hospital stay. It felt good to be able to be part of something which I knew and with which I was familiar. I still play, and it always soothes my spirit to hear the classical harmonies blend in my ears.

It was painful now to realize that maybe I would not be able to continue my medical studies. My doctor advised me not to study medicine. He said that it would be just too strenuous a lifestyle for me. He suggested I choose some other work that would not be quite so demanding. After some time, I decided that pharmacy might be a good choice.

Pharmacy Institute

In the fall, I applied to the Royal Institute of Pharmacy in Stockholm. (It later became the Division of Pharmacy at the University of Uppsala.) Prior to entering the technical course work of the Royal Institute of Pharmacy, I had to enlist in three years of practical work as a pharmaceutical apprentice. The reason being, I had to learn all the practical tasks and skills of a full-fledged pharmacist.

A Swedish pharmacy, which is called an *Apotek*, is very different from an American drug store. In those days, doctors in Sweden would prescribe pills and medications of specific strengths, and the pharmacist was expected to be able to formulate them to perfection in a timely manner, even though brand name drugs were available. The custom-made medications were prescribed by the doctor for patients with special needs. The pharmacist would make ointments, liniments, cough syrups, pills, salves, eye drops, etc. Many herbs, roots, barks and spices were used in preparing infusions and powders for natural, holistic preparations. At that time, fifteen to twenty percent of prescriptions needed this kind of preparation. Only after we were very skilled at weighing and mixing ingredients drop by drop on a scale were we allowed to make eye drops. They needed to be prepared in a sterile environment and then under strict supervision.

Since I enjoyed the protocols and detail of it all, I looked forward to the scientific coursework as well. The studies were extremely demanding, but I received my degree (similar to a Master's degree) and sat for the examination of the Royal Swedish Board of Pharmacy in Stockholm, to become a licensed and registered pharmacist, RPh, in 1963.

This was also the time in my life when I had to learn what it was like to live as a person with diabetes. *Symbiosis* is a term describing two entities that exist together, often to their mutual benefit. I believe that my pharmacy training and my diabetes training benefitted each other without my noticing it. Symbiosis – yes!

In my work at the pharmacy, I learned never to touch or lick a finger while mixing medicines. Even though some mixtures included flavorful ingredients, they could be very poisonous. That habit remains to this day. I rarely lick a finger when I am mixing anything in the kitchen, and that has saved me from eating extra carbohydrates and experiencing elevated blood sugar levels!

To this point, I had never known anybody else who had diabetes. One day, our landlord came to visit and my mother offered him a cup of coffee, and asked him whether he would like cream or sugar with it.

He said, "No thanks. I have my own sugar factory!"

Since there *was* a sugar factory in the neighboring town, I was impressed – "his own sugar factory"! – only to realize later that he was referring to himself. He was the first person I met with diabetes.

In 1964, I came to the United States to work for a year in diabetes research at the University of Minnesota. The insulin molecule had not yet been isolated. My job was to isolate and measure the amino acids in the insulin molecule found in cod pancreatic tissues, which included insulin. I used thin layer chromatography (of which I had achieved some expertise from my work at the Institute of Pharmacy). Some of this research was done under the leadership of Arnold Lazarow, MD, PhD (who would go on to receive the Banting Medal for Scientific Achievement Award in 1973).

During 1964, I got to know my friend, Vern Rice, who later proposed to me and gave me a diamond ring. He talked me into staying longer in Minnesota! It was a very exciting time. I was so happy to have found a wonderful man to marry, who loved me despite my diabetes and did not get hung up on the complications I *might* endure. Yet, I was wondering if health care in the United States would care for my diabetes as well as what I received in Sweden. (In Sweden all people with chronic illnesses get free medications and everything!)

I returned to Sweden to get ready for the wedding. It also was a bittersweet time: I was looking forward to a future full of fantastic possibilities, yet, was sad to leave my family and friends behind (with few chances to get together regularly). The wedding was held in *S Sallerup's church* in the countryside outside Malmö. The church was founded in 1160 AD; a white-washed structure of Danish architecture with three foot thick walls at the ground level. My father had been the pastor there for many years and was overjoyed that now he could perform the wedding for his daughter and son-in-law. I wore the gold bridal crown, which belonged to the church, and signed the record of brides who used that crown. The winters are mild in southern Sweden and we walked from the parsonage to the church (five minutes) in February, with snowdrop flowers blooming along the path. I remember grabbing a few caramels and eating them on the way, knowing how my blood sugar would often go low from the stress of excitement or having to perform; weddings are both!

After a few years, we were hoping to start a family. I worried about pregnancy and diabetes. My regimen was still one shot a day, without any change in urine testing. At the time, we did not live far from Rochester, Minnesota, where I knew I could get excellent pre-natal and diabetes care at the Mayo Clinic. With the excellent care there, I flourished! I had never felt so well in all my life.

I even had to cut down on my insulin dose as the baby's pancreas began to share its insulin with me, or so I thought at that time. (That is not possible, however, because mother's and baby's blood do not mix!) Current research has identified beta cell regeneration (an increase in the cells that produce insulin) in twenty percent of mothers with diabetes during the hormonal changes of pregnancy. I must have been one of those lucky ones and I felt great and was so thankful.

On the day that I was to be induced (two weeks early), I only administered four or six units of long-acting Lente insulin in the morning; my regular dose was about twenty-four units. After "my water broke," our son Jonathan was ready to be born. He was delivered within three hours, weighing in at 7 pounds, 13 ounces and measuring 21.5 inches long. A perfect size! My husband, Vern, said, "The joy of Jonathan's birth brought the widest smile I can ever remember to Birgitta's face!"

Even before Jonathan was born, we had discussed the size of our family. We had decided that we wanted to adopt a second child, primarily to avoid the risk of passing on diabetes, as Vern had diabetes in his family as well. A couple of years later, we adopted our daughter, Linnea, named for *Linnaea borealis* (Latin), which is commonly known in the United States as Twinflower; it's a small, fragrant, pink-flowered vine that grows both in the deep forests of Sweden as well as in northern Minnesota, Vern's home.

My diabetes routine continued for about twenty-two years with minor changes in dose of long-acting Lente insulin. Urine testing became easier when Tes-Tape® arrived in the 1970s, then testing became even easier with the introduction of blood glucose meters in the 1980s. What really threw me for a loop was changing the routine to twice-daily insulin shots. I was so upset with that change; I almost wanted to give up. I felt that it was almost worse than the very beginning of the disease. It was not that I had to take *more* insulin; actually I was splitting the dose into two. But I was unhappy that I had to give myself an extra shot each day!

As our children grew and I had more time, I became involved with the American Diabetes Association (ADA) and volunteered enthusiastically at both the local and regional levels. I even started thinking of becoming a diabetes educator. I had not been able to use my degree in pharmacy because of its foreign certification. It was almost impossible to get my degree accredited in America, which frustrated me. Yet I had so much knowledge and experience with diabetes. This spurred me on to go back to school. I had changed a bit and decided now to study for a Master's degree in Community Health Education at the University of Wisconsin – LaCrosse, and received an MS degree in 1990. I passed a national exam to become a Certified Health Education Specialist (CHES), which was a fairly new certification in 1990.

I had become more aware of what a person could accomplish using lifestyle changes and mind-body techniques to affect health and wellness, rather than focusing solely on pharmaceutical means. My scientific mind was challenged and my creative "right brain" mind flourished! I wondered, "Would there be any action that a person with diabetes could take that would help with complications in senior years?" I realized that most people have a motivation that drives them; mine was avoiding diabetes complications. The literature was full of scary examples of them. Regular exercise certainly would be good action to suggest – but that was not specific to diabetes; that is good for everyone!

As I studied stress management, I realized that, when learning the skill of relaxation, a person could affect the peripheral circulation. (The peripheral blood vessels in hands and feet widen, ever so little, and allow more blood to flow through them.) By first relaxing, then adding the mind-body method of visualizing warmth, you could imagine the feet feeling warmer and warmer, and so also see skin temperature rising with temperature biofeedback. This, without a doubt, became an exciting idea and the topic of my thesis research.

It was not going to be easy. The literature, at that time, also stated that people with diabetes were not good candidates for stress management, so in that sense, my hypothesis was questioned from the very start. But the outcome was significant! My research subjects with diabetes, both type 1 and type 2, ages seventeen to eighty-two years old, *all improved blood flow and temperature in their feet with relaxation training.* The findings of my study were later published in Diabetes Care, a medical journal of the American Diabetes Association; that gave my research wide publicity.

Research

I enjoyed this area of research and have worked on it both as an independent researcher, as well as at institutions, starting at the University of Wisconsin Medical School in Madison. In one of the studies, we used the same technique as earlier to measure what effect it would have on increasing the healing of chronic diabetic foot ulcers. Thirty-two patients with chronic foot ulcers were randomized into two groups. All got excellent wound care. The experimental group learned to improve blood flow using the relaxation technique; the control group did not. After twelve weeks, fourteen out of sixteen (87.5%) ulcers healed in the experimental group, while seven out of sixteen (43.75%) healed in the control group. Twice as many ulcers healed for those patients who learned to relax!

Of the nine patients who did not heal in the control group, five crossed over to learn the relaxation technique and were followed for an additional twelve weeks. Even though the five ulcers now were three months older at the start, they all healed – *all (100%) of them*! I was pretty pumped about that! Awards have been given for the *WarmFeet*® Intervention and I have had a chance to

181

speak to many national and international audiences. (See my Website for further information; it's listed at the end of my story.)

Here are some of the exciting results of my clinical work (two case studies).

1. A gentleman had signs of beginning gangrene and excruciating pain in his feet. He couldn't even eat or sleep. He learned the relaxation technique and in two weeks returned with increased blood flow and almost no pain. His scheduled amputation was put on hold and never executed.

2. A young man with a chronic non-healing heel ulcer learned the relaxation technique and after some time with the increased blood flow, his ulcer closed. When he returned to his vascular surgeon and reported the ulcer had healed, the technician responded: "We have no code for a healed heel ulcer!" I guess that is such an unusual occurrence that "a code" had never been established.

In the last fifteen years, I have again been working at the University of Minnesota. Currently the Epidemiology Clinical Research Center has been the home for my diabetes research. I'm involved with the National Institute of Diabetes and Digestive and Kidney Diseases-sponsored "Look AHEAD" (Action For Health in Diabetes) study, where we are looking for changes, using lifestyle modifications, to positively affect weight loss, cardiovascular and stroke risks in an obese population with type 2 diabetes. I also continue to write, consult, train and teach the technique now known as the *WarmFeet*® intervention. I am also available to interact and advise within the online diabetes community.

It is possible that my original wish to help seniors with diabetes is coming true. People who invest time in learning this natural, integrative, non-invasive *WarmFeet*® technique will realize its benefits: pain relief, increased healing, lower blood pressure, improved peripheral blood flow, and increased coping skills and wellness. This best happens when they also have good medical care and education.

My own diabetes regimen has evolved. I have, over the years, added more shots, up to four per day for a while, with combinations of different insulins. I keep tweaking my insulin/carbohydrate ratios also considering the effect of exercise and stress. Urine testing gave way to blood sugar monitoring many years ago. It indicates the blood glucose level right now; what a blessing! Diabetes education has also come a long way. Currently I am using the Animas Ping® insulin pump and I like it. When I started on the pump, I measured blood glucose as often as ten times a day.

Hypoglycemia has been my worst problem, and that has improved with the use of the pump. I hate the 3:00 AM "sweat-mares" that undo me for half a day. My husband helps me a great deal at night; at times, touching my forehead for signs of early perspiration and *hypoglycemia*. He has also brought me back, out of "the deep" *hypoglycemic* reactions, with the *glucagon* emergency kits. Otherwise, he lets me take care of myself without suggestions or prodding. I am so grateful to him. I have been fortunate in having very minor complications.

Fifteen years ago, I had open heart surgery to replace three blocked arteries. I had no symptoms before, nor after, the procedure. I decided to enter a six-month diet program to learn how to limit my saturated fat intake (in order to defy a repeat situation). However, I soon realized that I had used a very similar diet all along. I have pretty much maintained the same body measurements as I had when I was in high school.

When I reached the milestone of fifty years with diabetes, in 2009, I received the Joslin Gold Medal with the inscription: "Courageously Living with Diabetes 50 Years." I liked the way they worded that. I also decided to join the Joslin Gold Medal Longevity study, where they already have found some interesting results. For example, some of us in the "fifty year club" still have β-cells (beta cells) which produce precursors to insulin – after fifty years of diabetes!

In 2011, I visited my home town, Malmö, in Sweden and connected with a researcher at the Lund University hospital (the same place where my diabetes originally was diagnosed). He is leading the "PROLONG" diabetes study. They are inviting all people in Sweden with thirty years or more of diabetes duration to participate. They are looking for any measures or genes that PROmote the LONGevity with diabetes. Maybe a new remedy for diabetes will be discovered? Did I give them a sample of my blood? Yes; "you bet" as they say in Minnesota!

Last, but not least, my reason to title my chapter as I did. When I was growing up, my mother sewed most of my clothes. Since she was a very accomplished and creative seamstress, she could tailor me an outfit that I would not have been able to afford, and she enjoyed doing it. One time, she had a dreadful time getting the hem to hang straight. She didn't know if the fault was the weave of the fabric or how the pattern was cut, so she finally said: "Birgitta, you just have to walk fast and look happy!" We both burst out laughing. That advice has been precious to me in many different situations, diabetes notwithstanding.

Website: www.WarmFeetKit.com

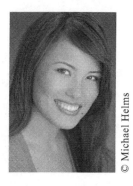
© Michael Helms

Chapter 18 *by Kyrra Richards*

A Diabetes Makeover

"I broke my bladder dancing in Afghanistan," I said to my doctor.

"Huh?" Apparently my doctor doubted my self-diagnosis.

I had just returned from a military tour, performing for the US troops in Afghanistan. As a twenty-four- year-old professional dancer working in Los Angeles, the opportunity was a nice change of pace from my usual commercial, music video, and award show gigs. The incredible experience had left me feeling grateful, fulfilled – and sick.

Ever since I had returned from my trip, I suffered from insatiable thirst. I ordered pitchers of water at restaurants and, in a single day, drank an entire tray of twenty-four water bottles. I'd race my young ballet students to the drinking fountain, and my sister began nicknaming me "Camel" as I'd loudly gulp my new Starbucks regular – "ice water – Venti."

Because I was drinking almost as much as an entire ocean, I spent most of my time in the bathroom. I'd make more-than-frequent pit stops on short drives and trudged to the toilet about five times per night between intense dreams of mystical lavatories. Exhausted and annoyed, I'd drag my zombie-like body down the hallway, doubting the logic of the term *rest*room.

I knew something had to be wrong, but my fear was overshadowed by delight for my noticeably trim figure. Each night as I danced the toilet tango, I weighed myself and observed the illuminated digits gradually decreasing. My brand new pair of jeans seemed surprisingly loose, two weeks after purchasing them, and it would hurt to sit for long periods of time as my bones protruded against seats. Even though I was aware that my ribs were becoming more visible, I was booking jobs one after another – concert dance performances and international print campaigns. Stylists had fun dressing me in high-end couture and complimented me on my tiny legs. Choreographers would use me as the demonstration subject for partner lifts, and photographers would have male models pick me up as we posed in fashion shoots. My career was taking off.

At first, I attributed the weight loss to my busy schedule and dedicated workout regimen. I danced each day for hours and ate healthily. It seemed only right that my body was changing.

But was it changing too fast?

I would sit and contemplate the negative possibilities of my condition – a tape worm? A tumor? Thyroid problems? After reevaluating my past actions, I decided the most logical conclusion was that I had damaged my bladder after forcing myself to "hold it" as I traveled between Afghanistan bases in military planes. The soldiers would announce before takeoff, "Ladies, if you need to go, you are welcome to use this bucket here. There are no separate bathrooms on these flights."

I opted to hold it.

I knew I needed to see a doctor, but I didn't want to risk losing my thin figure and professional success as I endured a surgery that would require the worst prescription for a dancer – rest. I decided to ignore my intuition.

It wasn't until a close friend met me for frozen yogurt and worriedly commented about my weight loss that I knew I needed more than a standard checkup. I called to schedule an appointment. In my gut, I knew the visit would not be so "standard."

I proceeded with my damaged bladder explanation despite my doctor's stunned expression. After listening and responding with a "Hmmm . . ." she requested my response to a few additional questions.

"Have you been abnormally hungry lately?" she asked.

"Always. I love to eat," I told her.

"Have you been extremely thirsty?"

"Definitely!"

"Have you been feeling tired?"

"Who hasn't?"

"Uh . . . huh . . . I'm going to need a couple more tests to verify the problem, but I have a good idea. I'm going to have a nurse come in and do a simple blood test by pricking your finger."

"Okay," I replied.

"And then I'll need a urine test," she said.

"That won't be difficult," I replied wryly.

After I returned from yet another trip to the restroom, a young nurse came in to follow the doctor's orders. She spoke to me casually as she pricked my finger and dropped the blood onto a tiny mechanism of a small machine. As she looked down to read the screen on the device, her eyes grew very wide and she stopped mid-sentence.

"What? Is it bad?" Nothing could be good based on *that* expression.

"Um . . . I'll have the doctor come right in."

That wasn't a good sign. I began to panic. After the most traumatic few minutes of my life, the doctor entered to look at my results. Her eyebrows automatically lifted and then she let out a big sigh.

"Unfortunately, it's just as I suspected. Honey, you have diabetes."

Now, if I could write this next part of the story in slow motion, it would be a more adequate way of describing my heart-wrenching, breathless, and inexplicably confused state as I sat frozen on the exam table.

My doctor calmly continued with, "You have all the textbook signs, Kyrra. I hardly needed to take this test, but your blood sugar level is at 497 mg/dL."

I remember thinking, *Okay . . . what does that mean? Am I going to die?*

But my doctor hadn't finished speaking. She said, "An average, healthy reading is anywhere from 80 mg/dL to 110 mg/dL or so. It's a good thing that you came into the office today; otherwise, you may have ended up in a coma. We need to get you straight to the hospital to see an endocrinologist and get your blood sugar down immediately."

"But I'm supposed to work in a few hours. I need to go over choreography with my students for our upcoming show."

"Honey, you're very sick. You need to call your boss and tell her that you can't dance. We need to take care of this matter right away – you're in a very dangerous state. I'll be back in a few minutes." She closed the door.

That's it? Just like that? No debate? Surely, she had to be mistaken. My life was a constant battle for perfection – I was repeatedly honored on the Dean's List, captain of the UCLA cheerleading team, selected by the top dance agency in Hollywood, and would do fifty-one sit-ups in training sessions, if fifty were required. I couldn't accept weakness.

As the severity of her words set in, I couldn't stop the stream of tears as they poured down my face, still frozen from shock. I was a strong, independent young woman who took pride in controlling her own life. For the very first time, I felt completely helpless.

The next few weeks were a blur – endless doctor appointments, countless hours in waiting rooms, and listless nights as tears soaked my pillow. I was no longer a dancer. I was a patient. I had been diagnosed with type 1 diabetes. Even though my age countered the widely-used "juvenile" diabetes term, I felt childlike and immature as I took my first steps into this new lifestyle. Even my initial endocrinologist made it seem as though I had skipped an obvious training session due to my abnormally late diagnosis of diabetes.

"So, you have diabetes," she said. "Don't worry – a lot of famous people have diabetes."

Oh, well, I thought. *In that case, bring on the damaged pancreas. At least I'll get to be in US Weekly!*

"Just go home and give yourself a shot of insulin and come back tomorrow," she said. "Your blood sugar numbers should go down."

Wait, is she talking to me? She must mean the nurse. The nurse has to give me a shot of something? I looked around. "Um . . . a shot of what?"

Exasperated, she repeated, "Give yourself a shot of insulin!"

I stared back in silence. Had I somehow missed the lesson on self-inflicting insulin shots in freshman health class? After she finally stopped staring at my file, she looked up and noticed my awkward reaction.

"Wait, you don't know how to give yourself a shot of insulin?"

Oh, I must have forgotten – I actually won the gold medal in insulin-shooting, I thought sarcastically.

"No. I just found out I have diabetes an hour ago. I don't even really understand what that means."

"Ugh – hold on." She opened the door and stuck her head out to scream to a nurse down the hall, "Patty, get in here – she doesn't even know how to give herself a shot of insulin!"

(I no longer see that endocrinologist.)

Act Two of my life had begun. I was given new choreography to learn – constant prancing to the hospital, frequent turns to the diabetes educator's office, continuous curtsies to the pharmacy, and extremely long intermissions in waiting rooms. And because I was beginning to feel like an understudy to my former self, I was sent to a therapist specializing in chronic illness.

"So how do you feel today?" The therapist asked in a soothing tone.

"Awful," I replied.

"And why is that?"

"Well, I was propelled into a medical lifestyle that requires me to inject a foreign liquid into my body that causes me to gain weight like Santa Claus. It severely affects my ability to work as a professional dancer. I'm not allowed to exercise heavily until my blood sugar numbers go down, so I get to stare at a funhouse mirror reflection while my confidence and bank account plummet. I've handed over most of my modeling earnings to the pharmacist and have started valuing objects in terms of diabetes supplies – my dinner tonight cost about thirty-six test strips."

I went on with, "While the insulin may aid the nourishment of my body, it has not filled my hungry mentality. I can't help my natural inclination to eat constantly, but then feel extreme guilt and anger as I contribute to my weight gain. After using insulin to correct the high glucose levels from my binges, I often plunge into dangerous *hypoglycemia* and restart the entire stressful cycle as I walk the midnight pathway toward the refrigerator. I feel unattractive – physically and professionally, and lay awake at night, longing for my former, ignorant lifestyle. I'm a mess."

The therapist listened calmly, and tried to reassure me with kind, empathetic words. While I appreciated her attempts to help, after a few more sessions I decided I could not afford my expensive rants. I thanked her, excused myself, and didn't return.

I received her bill and conclusive paperwork in the mail a week later – a crisp, white form with my diagnosis clearly labeled: "depression."

No kidding, I thought. *This painfully obvious diagnosis just cost me 1400 units of insulin.*

I was trapped in a muted, medical maze and spent countless hours in an austere hospital environment. My world was compromised by my dejected outlook, and I felt as though my condition was apparent to everyone. To make matters worse, I was forced to carry around my essential diabetes tools in a drab nylon case.

You might as well stick a nametag on my forehead – 'Hello, my name is SICK.'

I hated its medicinal appearance and would often "forget" to pack the dingy case as I raced off to lunch. The bland case just didn't complement my trendy, colorful purse – diabetes was clashing with my lifestyle.

My insecurities were obvious when I met up with friends for dinner. After ordering the low-carbohydrate option, I subtly reached into my purse for my testing supplies. I needed to draw a blood droplet from my finger and check my sugar levels before eating, so I carefully unzipped the little black case underneath the table and laid it on my knees. I was embarrassed and didn't want to draw attention to my abnormality.

As I nervously waited for my blood sugar results, I happened to glance across the restaurant aisle and notice an all-too-familiar scene. An older man sitting at the next table reached into his pocket to expose an identical nylon case. He discreetly placed it on his lap and continued his own glucose testing process.

All of a sudden, I realized that this stranger was suffering from the same ridiculous set of diabetic social issues. Clearly, we were two distinct individuals, yet the same shoddy case was positioned on my purple dress and his khaki slacks. Why were we both pitifully hiding the same standard-issue supply kit? We were from different generations. We had different evening plans. We had ordered different meals. So why were we distributed the same sterile bag? Where was the medical menu? We needed to *choose* our diabetes styles.

I returned home, renewed by my revelation. I grabbed a plain white sheet of paper and started to draft my ideas to change the homogeneous health industry. My pen flew across the page. I drew cases in various shapes, fabrics, and colors specifically for glucose meters, lancing devices, and insulin pumps. I sketched wallets, belts, and purses suitable for the pages of *Diabetic Vogue*. I was going to give diabetes a well-needed makeover.

189

My favorite design was heartfelt and personal. I thought about my days spent in rigid hospital laboratories and doctors' offices. They were hard for me to tolerate, but what if my young students had been thrown into this grueling regimen? I typically spent my afternoons with toddlers in tutus, using creative imagery to teach basic ballet. My little girls loved frilly, descriptive language – pink, purple, shiny, sparkly, polka-dotted, magical – words perfect for princesses. The diabetes process, however, was certainly not a royal experience.

I decided to create a special case that my young ballerinas would love. I carefully crafted a heart-shaped bag that opened to reveal a colorful butterfly inside. I drew elastic loops and pockets along the butterfly's wings to store testing necessities. I even added a smile to the little bug so that kids would be greeted by a friendly face when they needed to prick their fingers. I wanted to make the experience more fun and develop responsible habits by associating the routine with positive images.

For the first time in months, I felt energized. My happy butterfly and fashionable designs would help improve the diabetes routine. Instead of apathetically surrendering to the disease, I could contribute.

But now what? I had a good idea, but how was I going to implement it? I was a planner, and a diabetes design company certainly wasn't on my original life list. I wasn't prepared. I had no experience; my academic and performance resume had no trace of medical fashion practice. I had no savings; the pharmacy had seized practically all my assets. It seemed like such an enormous responsibility – changing the entire outlook of an established health community. I wasn't sure I had the courage to bear another battle. The months of despondency had worn me down. I decided to put my style revolution on hold. I stashed my secret sketches deep in the filing cabinet and closed the drawer. I'd claim my plans another day.

Months passed with the same struggle and tedious testing. It was a constant adjustment, and life as an auditioning dancer added more anxiety. Every day I was asked by a casting office to fill out a statistics sheet – Weight? Measurements – bust, waist, hips? Dress size? Pant size? These simple questions seemed to be directed toward my insecurities.

I thought in response, *Is there a space for an explanation? Maybe a "diabetes" box to check?*

I'd then be called into the casting room to begin the audition process. It was always the same routine:

"Please stand on the X in the center of the room and look straight toward the camera."

I'd place my toes along the tape lines and, to disguise my fear, focus my eyes firmly forward.

"Name?"

"Hi, my name is Kyrra Richards," I asserted with a grin.

"Profiles."

I'd turn to the right, hold up my hair to expose all features of my neck and face then repeat with the other side. I'd then wait for the next dreaded words.

"Slow 360."

This was my recurring nightmare. I'd hold my breath and pivot toward the back wall. I'd pause as they studied my rear side and then pivot again to face the camera. Then I'd think, *Were they laughing? Were they going to dismiss me immediately? Did the fifteen additional pounds appear to be thirty in the camera?* This slating process, a critical part of the casting process, was a relentless mind game.

"Hands."

This was my cue to hold up both hands and flip them back and forth. The directors wanted to make sure their models and dancers had all ten fingers in case they had to be filmed holding a product. This final casting requirement used to be the easy part of auditions, but now I was nervous that they would notice the little calluses and scars on my fingers from testing six times a day.

They would eventually turn on music and instruct me to dance in front of the camera for nearly a minute. My job was all about aesthetics. Did I fit the role description? Could I fit into the clothing samples? Did I have the right color hair? What was my ethnic appearance? Were my proportions appealing? Was I the right look for their project?

These questions didn't disappear after I left castings. They incessantly dominated my thoughts, diminishing my self-worth. *Was I the right look?* The industry's rejection was difficult, but my own judgment was far worse. My physical appearance had control of my career, but diabetes had control over my physicality. My pancreas had given its two-week notice and caused my livelihood to suffer.

Hollywood's aesthetic authority was clearly displayed one afternoon during a standard commercial audition. I waited for my turn in the lobby with my headshot in-hand. After ten minutes, they called my name and instructed me to stand on the familiar X on the casting studio floor. The casting director and his assistants were seated on a black, leather couch at the end of the room. I greeted them with a cheerful hello and took my place center stage. The director held up one finger to pause my audition and reached into his pocket to answer his cell phone. Soon his brow furrowed, and he began shouting. In my little dress and heels, I stood uncomfortably as, for the next several minutes, he continued his loud, public fight.

When he finally hung up, he shook his head and looked at me. "Excuse me hun, just dealing with some work issues."

"No problem." I answered casually despite my discomfort.

"See, you don't have to deal with this stuff."

"Oh, yeah?" I asked.

"Yeah. You're pretty, so you don't have to use your brain."

After that, I only remember the instant paralysis and astonishment. His ignorant statement pierced through my defensive shield and caused my sugary blood to boil. I was an educated, accomplished young woman with big dreams and well-tested tenacity. Why was I allowing myself to be subjected by this demeaning, egotistical executive? And even more importantly, why was I searching for approval and validation from these outside sources?

I stormed out of the studio with a new mission. I needed to shift my mindset and regain my self-worth. I couldn't let diabetes and its unexpected tribulations call the shots; I needed to fight. My passion had been dormant long enough. Pre-diagnosis, I had believed that I was on the path to something special. I was destined to live an extraordinary life. The past year, however, had forced me to question my originality. I felt lonely and ordinary. I had been bar-coded and stocked on the sugar-free shelf. "Diabetes" had become my identity. Now it was time to strip this label and reclaim my individuality. Life may have cast me in this role, but now I was going to demand the spotlight.

The day of change had arrived. I pulled out my sketches and began devising a plan to create a diabetes accessory company. I gathered my most brilliant, successful friends with backgrounds in marketing, finance and law. Their talent and empathetic energy created the perfect founding team to execute my vision. As administrative tasks began to fall into place, we needed to clarify our purpose with a powerful brand. If I was going to re-label my new outlook, it needed to be compelling.

I sat on my bed with a clean notepad and began jotting down every diabetes-related name I could imagine.

Diabetter . . . DiaCouture . . . Design-a-betic . . .

I needed an inclusive moniker that represented the distinct, personal aspect of a lifestyle with diabetes. I decided to switch techniques and, instead, write down my own goals for a diabetes transformation. Why was I adopting a new attitude? What inspired me to persist?

My family
My students
My career
My goals
My dreams
My legacy

Suddenly, it was obvious. Diabetes didn't define me. It was a part of my life, but not my entire identity. I would manage my health the same way I manage every other aspect of my life – with my personal style.

My life. My health. My style. MYabetic.

Myabetic was founded with a vision for change. It was time to end the impersonal, standard-issue criterion for diabetes care. I wanted better, more vibrant options. Apparently, I was not alone.

Men, women, and children from all over the world began to purchase our Myabetic products. They ordered wallets, cases, purses, and accessories in various colors and fabrics. They wanted diversity. They wanted to embrace their unique qualities. They shared my vision.

Starting a company was quite an adventure. Like my glucose levels, it was a series of highs and lows. I worried as I waited for our very first prototypes to arrive. *What if the designs weren't perfect? What if they weren't how I'd envisioned? What if they couldn't improve the negative stigma associated with diabetes?*

But after apprehensively opening the first box, I unwrapped a familiar-looking object and knew we had started something special. I picked up the pink, heart-shaped case and unzipped it to find a colorful butterfly smiling back at me. My "Love Bug" had arrived.

Months later, I was sent a video of an adorable kindergartener receiving her new Love Bug case. After inserting her diabetes supplies into the proper pockets and loops, she hugged it to her chest and proclaimed, "This is my most favorite thing in the world!" Tears welled up as I realized my dream was coming true.

Diabetes is still challenging and unpredictable. There are still days I wish I could trade my busted pancreas for a damaged bladder, but I've learned to accept imperfection and endure life's unexpected turns. This particular hiccup inspired me to build a company and become part of the amazingly supportive diabetes community. Their overwhelming enthusiasm reinforces my drive to succeed.

My diabetes diagnosis changed my life path, but it didn't change my purpose. I was meant to do something special – make over the medical world. Instead of settling for something mundane, we can demand higher standards and options that reflect our individuality. I have diabetes, but I can still perform, create, and educate while maintaining healthy habits. I can use my artistic passion to promote positivity and inspire others to face their diabetes with determination and optimism. That's *my* style.

Website: www.myabetic.com

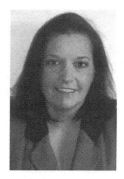

Chapter 19   *by Lisa Ritchie*

Diabetes: Not Just a Diagnosis - It's a Lifestyle

Since the age of eleven, I've had to live with an incurable disease that affects every single aspect of my life. No one knows I have it, unless I tell them, because type 1 diabetes is not visible or obvious. I can never take a vacation from it or ignore it. I must plan my every move in advance: what I will eat, when I will be eating, and how much activity I will be doing. I must always carry my medication and testing supplies with me. I also face the possibility of serious, debilitating complications.

The Diagnosis: The Early Years

At age eleven, despite a healthy diet, I was rapidly losing weight. When I reached only seventy-nine pounds, my mother became increasingly concerned. She wanted me to go to the doctor. I felt that I was too old to sit in the waiting room of my pediatrician with crying infants, so we chose a local physician. Unfortunately, I was misdiagnosed as a person with type 2 diabetes.

My parents and I were not aware of any incidence of diabetes in my family history. I was only eleven years old and didn't realize how serious the situation was. I just did what I was told. At first, I was treated as a type 2 patient with oral medication, diet, and exercise. This type of treatment was completely the wrong protocol for me, a person with type 1 diabetes. I should have been started on insulin injections immediately.

In addition, this was in the early 1970s and in-home testing was only via urine samples. Essentially, test results were based on actions that had taken place hours before. Today, there are blood glucose testing meters to monitor your blood sugar levels, which provide much more accurate results, as these give an immediate reading of one's blood sugar. How times have changed!

But when I was diagnosed, it was in the early 1970s. While the method of treatment I was being given did keep my blood sugar levels within a normal range, I was not gaining weight, nor did I have the energy that an eleven-year-old should have.

After six months of little progress in my health, my parents brought me back to my original pediatrician. He took one look at me and immediately admitted me to the hospital for ten days. It was then that I was actually diagnosed with type 1 diabetes, which, at the time, was referred to as "juvenile diabetes." I was put on insulin, which was made from beef and/or pork. The hospital staff taught me how to administer injections to myself. I was taught to inject my insulin under the skin thirty minutes before a meal (which wasn't always easy to plan for). This allowed the insulin enough time to peak in effectiveness in order to cover the carbohydrates eaten at each meal.

After I left the hospital, I remember struggling emotionally to insert the needle into my thigh. It didn't really hurt, but in my mind I couldn't slip it in slowly or gently enough. It would take me twenty to thirty minutes to complete one injection. Today I do it so quickly and easily it's second nature.

I also had to endure a day-long test - the glucose tolerance test – which involved drinking regular Coca-Cola® and having my blood drawn at specific intervals. It was a laborious affair and excruciating for an eleven-year-old. Today, testing methods have greatly improved with the A1C test, which measures the amount of sugar that has attached to proteins (red blood cells) over the course of three months. It can be done any time of the day without fasting. There is even an "at home" version (which is not a substitute for having an A1C test done at a physician's office).

One positive outcome from all this blood testing was the discovery that I am a carrier of Cooley's anemia. It's a genetic illness that could be fatal if it was passed down to my child, and this influenced my decision not to have children. I'm glad I found out!

I didn't know anyone who had type 1 diabetes, and I felt frustrated, because I had no one to relate to, or to ask questions of. I felt entirely alone. I was uneducated about what was happening to me, and I couldn't understand the seriousness of the disease. There were no advocacy groups or organized meetings that I knew of in my area. There wasn't even the Internet back then to do my own research!

My parents and my older sister couldn't relate to what I was going through. As I got older, both my mother and maternal grandmother were diagnosed with type 2 diabetes, a different pathology of the disease.

My parents always took good care of me: made my meals, made sure I tested my urine and took my shots. But from the beginning, I have always given myself my own injections. In the beginning, I was mixing a set dosage of long-acting insulin (NPH) with a morning dose of short-acting insulin (Regular) once a day, without any adjustments.

I started gaining some weight back and started coping with life on insulin. I went to school, participated in theatre and other clubs, and took my shot before breakfast, thereby eliminating the need to carry my supplies with me. Looking back, it was like "shooting in the dark."

I recall once, when I was in the seventh grade, I had a low blood sugar reaction. I remember it vividly. I was in Social Studies class and suddenly felt dizzy. I stood up to be excused to go to the nurse's office and made it out into the hallway, where I passed out – right into the arms of the most popular boy in school, who happened to be passing by. How embarrassing! He managed to get the nurse, who gave me some orange juice. I was mortified. This instilled in me a deep paranoia about having medical problems in public.

The Teenage Years

I stayed active as a teenager. I joined the track team in junior high school and went roller skating every weekend. I had a small rowboat that I used on the river behind our home. I always got into the habit, though, of carrying small packets of sugar or jellybeans in my pocket at all times. (This was before the days of cell phones.) I never wanted to pass out from *hypoglycemia* again, and this fear has stayed with me even to this day. As a result, my blood sugars tend to average slightly higher than recommended, much to my doctor's dismay.

I never made my diabetes an issue, but all my closest friends knew about it just in case anything should happen and I needed help. I simply went about my daily routine without a second thought as to the seriousness of this disease. I dated, and the topic never seemed to come up. At that age, we went roller skating or to concerts, rather than out to dinner, so taking an injection never came into the picture. I remained very active: cycling, walking and going out in my rowboat with my friends, which helped control my blood sugar levels.

Eventually, my insulin regimen increased to taking the mixed shot in the morning, plus another dose of Regular insulin before dinner. Some years later, I added a third shot at lunch time, now covering each meal with a separate injection of short-acting insulin.

197

College

I decided to go away to college, perhaps not the best decision in retrospect. I chose a school in southern Virginia, and I was looking forward to my independence.

Emotionally, this is when the diabetes hit me like a ton of bricks. Suddenly, my parents weren't there to oversee my meals and make sure I did the right things. (If I didn't tell you, you simply wouldn't know that I had diabetes.) I drank alcohol and stayed out late. I ate all the "wrong" foods. I was in complete denial. I took full advantage of my new freedom.

At one point, I caught the flu. I was dehydrated and delirious. My roommates physically picked me up and drove me to the local hospital. I was immediately put on an intravenous drip. It was very traumatic for me because I didn't have my own doctor or family nearby. I recovered within a week and returned to classes.

At first, I majored in English Education and then changed to Print Journalism. I discovered the campus radio station and finally decided on my chosen career. Unfortunately, I discovered my love for broadcasting *after* I had decided to move back to New York, leaving my degree unfinished. I did well for the first few months back home, working at various office jobs in order to save enough money to go back to school and break into the broadcasting industry.

Post-College

I started to recognize the reality of my disease. I had already gone through the denial phase. Now I moved on to anger, resentment and depression. I thought, *Why me? Why was I chosen for this disease; what had I done?* I thought about reincarnation. Was this punishment for something I'd done in a previous life? Was this some sort of karmic challenge from the Universe?

Diabetes educators weren't available yet and I had no one to talk to who understood my issues. The only support groups I could locate were designed for very young children with diabetes. I still don't know why I was chosen to have type 1 diabetes.

In my early twenties, I went from denial – in effect, ignoring my disease – to obsession, dwelling too much on my diabetes. I worried about passing out in public and whether anyone would know what to do. When blood testing meters became available, I owned several, including one that was pocket-sized. I constantly checked my blood sugar. My doctor recommended testing before each meal and before bed, but I tested up to *twenty or thirty times* a day! My fingertips were sore with calluses, yet I *had* to know what my number was. I became so consumed with my diabetes that I developed *agoraphobia*.

I lost several office jobs as my anxiety attacks increased in frequency and severity. I was constantly leaving work early or calling out sick. Eventually, my parents found out and then I would stay home in my bedroom, feeling miserable and useless. My endocrinologist recommended a psychiatrist whom I just didn't connect with. She was too Freudian, when all my problems were anxiety-based over my diabetes. I quit after a few sessions. I then found a clinical social worker. We hit it off right away. She was more understanding, methodical and encouraging.

I started my therapy by walking outside to the front porch every day. This took all of my concentration as the anxiety overwhelmed me. The following week I would go to the mailbox. Eventually, I was walking around the block (though always loaded down with my jellybeans and blood test meter). She told me if I felt the need to test, to go ahead: test my blood sugar, my temperature, my pulse, my blood pressure, and anything else that would reassure me that everything was fine. After awhile, I learned that these were physical manifestations, created by my mind, and that I could control them.

Adulthood

Eventually, I overcame the *agoraphobia* and panic attacks. I successfully enrolled in a local community college and graduated with a degree in Broadcast Telecommunications, earning an internship at the number-one rated radio station on Long Island. In my final semester, I was offered a job producing the morning show. I jumped at it and still managed to graduate on the Dean's List. The County Executive was the keynote speaker at my graduation, the same man who I'd interviewed just that morning!

I not only overcame my anxiety and *agoraphobia*, but eventually I became a local "broadcast personality." After over twenty-five years as a radio disc jockey, news reporter and morning show producer, I am also currently employed full-time as an on-air traffic reporter for a regional cable television network in the New York Tri-state area. My job requires me to make public appearances, go on stage and introduce bands and celebrities, attend press conferences, and interact with politicians and community leaders.

I realized that by always being prepared, there was no need to fear any circumstances. I also realized that my body gives off its own warning signals. When my blood sugar falls too low, my left outer thigh will "tingle." I became adept at sensing it. People who knew me during my anxiety attack phase can't believe how confident and outgoing I've become. I'm quite a "ham."

I've also become quite a highly organized planner. I am like a Boy Scout – always prepared! To this day, I make sure that I always have my meter, test strips, and sugar packets or jellybeans for emergencies. In addition to my insulin and syringes, I also pack all my meals for the day into a small cooler. There are times that my job requires me to stay overnight in a hotel on the spur of the moment, and I'm always glad I have all my supplies handy.

I now realize that while type 1 diabetes is inconvenient, with some planning, I can live well with it. There are plenty of other diseases in the world that are more difficult (or fatal). Having my supplies ready helps, though it does prevent me from carrying a small purse!

Clinical Research Trials

I've participated in two clinical trials conducted by a highly reputable research center. Each was held for one full year, during which time all my supplies and testing were paid for. The first clinical research trial was for a very rapid-acting injectable insulin. I loved it! This drug allows you to eat *first* and take your injection immediately *after* your meal. This allowed for a great deal more freedom and flexibility in meal planning. My blood sugar levels remained in their typical range (for me) and I had no side effects. Sadly, I never heard that the insulin made it to market.

The second clinical research trial was for a powdered, inhaled insulin. I hated it! My throat was sore all the time, and the drug was administered in tiny vials through a plastic pipe. This was somewhat embarrassing, and not very subtle to take in public. I also found that a tremendous amount of insulin would have to be inhaled for it to be effective. My blood sugar levels seemed sky high for the entire year of the trial. Luckily, constant testing was being done for my kidneys, eyes, and lungs to check for side effects.

This trial was held post-September 11, 2001, but I was amazed when I flew to Florida from New York and back. No one questioned the unmarked vials filled with white powder in my carry-on luggage. The only place that asked me about it was at the Kennedy Space Center!

Complications

I haven't always been the ideal patient, but I'm lucky enough not to have developed any major complications (yet). However, I was diagnosed with *diabetes-exacerbated periodontal disease*. It all started when I was eight years old and fell off my bicycle, knocking out one of two front teeth. The orthodontist at the time re-implanted the tooth (root and all) and put braces on to hold it in place. It attached, but unfortunately, fused to the bone and never grew. Eventually that tooth was removed and I wore a plastic plate with a tooth attached until my mouth stopped growing. At that point, I was fitted with a bridge. But, due to the periodontal disease, the bridge kept coming loose; the teeth underneath it were rotting. I would go through four different bridges, each one becoming wider and wider and damaging more teeth underneath.

At age forty-four, I decided to investigate dental implant surgery. It was emotionally very traumatic, as I was toying with my livelihood as an on-air announcer, where I speak for a living. I was very upset by several doctors' opinions, as each of them came to the same conclusion: remove all my upper teeth! *What?* I seriously had to consider the repercussions of taking, or not taking, this route. I chose an excellent surgeon who used CAT-scan technology to measure my mouth, locate all the nerves, etc., and used general anesthesia for the surgeries. I decided to follow the doctors' recommendation and had *all* of my remaining upper teeth removed; the surgeon inserted nine dental implants.

The entire process took over two years, as the surgery was done in two stages to avoid the use of dentures. Once the implants took hold in the jaw bone, the crowns would be perfectly fitted to match the bottom teeth, so that the bite would be correct and the color and length would match, as well. (They are now my "bionic" teeth.) It was a very pricey procedure, but well worth it. They look natural and are very comfortable, and unlike dentures, are permanent. They have not affected my speech.

In 2010, I was diagnosed with borderline *high blood pressure*, approximately 140/70. I tried a low-dose medication which I developed an allergy to, so I am now controlling my blood pressure through diet, exercise and stress reduction.

Also in 2010, my ophthalmologist discovered two tiny vessels bleeding in my retina; the start of *retinopathy*. He sent me to a specialist, who informed me that the ruptures were so tiny that I shouldn't worry about them, but to control my blood sugar levels, avoid strenuous lifting, and revisit the doctor in six months. At that follow-up visit, my doctor told me they had healed and everything was okay. What a relief!

Also in 2010, I discovered a rather odd side effect. I'm afflicted with *hives*. Apparently it is a condition that occurs in people with autoimmune diseases. There is no cure, but it can be treated with high doses of antihistamines. I discovered by accident that one of those medications caused a reduction in blood sugar levels. I was wondering why my readings were suddenly so low, because I was eating the same foods and taking the same insulin dose. After some Internet research, I discovered that the prescription strength version of Allegra® caused the drop in my blood sugar. As a result, I adjusted my insulin dose.

The *hives* seem to come and go. Now that I think back on it, I've had this since my teen years but I always assumed it was a skin allergy. It was only when it became stubborn and wouldn't go away that I discovered its true cause.

Technology and the Future

I am still hesitant to move forward with the latest technology. I do not want to wear an insulin pump or even a continuous glucose monitor (CGM). As I write this, I've lived with insulin-dependent diabetes for thirty-nine years. Today, I take two separate shots in the morning before breakfast (short-acting Humalog®, which is a recombinant human DNA insulin, and Lantus®, a "peakless" insulin, to cover my day). I also take Humalog® at both lunch and dinner, and "shorter" long-acting NPH insulin before bed to cover me through the night, making a total of five shots a day. I prefer my insulin injections and finger sticks to test my blood; I'm used to it and it doesn't bother me. But I keep hoping islet cell transplants or a true "cure" will be found.

Active Athletic Lifestyle

Toward that goal of finding a cure, I am currently involved in doing charity work for the Juvenile Diabetes Research Foundation, marketing fundraising events, and advocacy in an effort to support the development of a cure. Exciting research is being done with regards to islet cell transplants and fighting rejection. In 2007, I single-handedly raised over $1,500.00 for the American Diabetes Association's "Tour de Cure" cycling event, a thirty-six mile bike tour, proving that a person with type 1 diabetes can lead an active, athletic life with proper planning.

In 1993, I earned my National Certification as a Personal Fitness Trainer through ACE, the American Council on Exercise. In addition to the full-time work on cable television, I also run my own personal fitness training business, specializing in women's fitness. I occasionally lecture about fitness and healthy living to corporate and civic groups. I'm also a freelance writer for an Internet wellness website. I exercise daily and I'm an avid road cyclist. In colder months, I train indoors on my own Spinning® bike and lift weights. In the summer, I swim, road bike and continue to do strength workouts. I've always said, "When they find the cure, I'll be the healthiest person alive!"

A Positive Attitude

Living with type 1 diabetes certainly isn't easy and comes with its own challenges, but I look at each challenge as an opportunity for growth and a new learning experience. (How boring would life be without challenges?) Every day is different, and blood sugar levels can fluctuate. You must become adept at adjusting insulin, activity levels, and meals. Many times it feels like a tight-rope walk!

Most of all, it is important to understand diabetes and accept it. It is treatable and I *can* live a successful life with it, if I take care of myself. Along with exercise and healthy eating, blood sugar testing is crucial to keeping blood sugar levels within a target range. I try to be a proactive patient, ask questions, get second and third opinions, and educate myself as much as possible.

I often think about the silver lining of being diagnosed as a person with type 1 diabetes. It has made me resourceful, responsible and independent. I have become a very thorough planner. I'm a great cook and eat healthy "clean" meals with as little processed food as possible. (In other words, I don't see myself reaching for a piece of double fudge cake when [not if!] a cure for diabetes is found.)

Most of all, it has led me to live a very healthy life, as diabetes is not just a diagnosis. It's a lifestyle. Sure, I have "up" days and "down" days, but I always remind myself that there is no time like the present to turn it around. You have two choices: a negative attitude, or a positive attitude. I find that being positive reaps greater rewards.

Website: www.health4her.webs.com

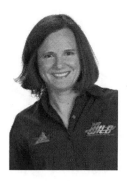

Chapter 20 *by Mari Ruddy, MA*

Taking Control of One's Diabetes Health through Athletics

I like to travel and have adventures. When I first learned to walk, I took myself immediately over to the neighbor's house to see what was going on! I kept my parents on their toes. Now, as an adult, my work takes me all over the United States almost on a weekly basis. I like meeting people, moving around and bringing people together. When I was a kid, I liked to get everybody on the block together and make forts and put on plays. My parents were adventurous, too, and we went camping and hiking often. We didn't have a lot of money, but my mom and dad knew how to use their imaginations and create a lot of fun spending very little cash. They were creative.

All of our family vacations didn't go smoothly, however. That's because, in the late 1960's and 1970's, blood glucose testing wasn't yet available, except in the lab. When I was one year old, my dad, who was 26 years old, was diagnosed with type 1 diabetes. He couldn't always predict when his blood sugar would suddenly drop from the hiking or canoeing. My dad is a big guy, 6 feet 4 inches and over 200 pounds., and when he had a bad low, he tended toward convulsions and going unconscious. It was scary beyond measure. My mom couldn't always see the warning signs in time to get orange juice and sugar into him fast enough. When that was the case, she called the paramedics. Each time it happened, which was about once a year, my brother, sister and I stood together watching and crying and wondering if *this* time, he would die.

This early imprint of what diabetes was and how it could impact those around you has affected my entire life. And it made June 26, 1981, an especially poignant day in my own life. I was sixteen, and it was just after the 10th grade had let out for the summer. I started to lose weight and I was thirsty all the time and, of course, I had to urinate every fifteen minutes (it seemed). You guessed it, and so did my mom and dad. We had the Tes-Tape® because of my dad's diabetes. I urinated on it and, sure enough, it turned the darkest green possible.

It was the evening and we knew, because we knew about diabetes, that it could wait until the morning for me to go to the clinic. My dad and I sat on the couch for a long time together and cried. He kept saying he was so sorry. I kept trying to reassure him that I would be okay. I was trying to reassure myself, too, that I would be okay. Even though I had my dad, who understood, I still remember how lost and alone I felt. And I never wanted to scare the people around me the way I was scared of his diabetes. I didn't know how I would be able to do that, but I resolved to figure it out, if I could.

When we went in the next day, the pediatrician told us my blood sugar was 350 mg/dL, which was bad, but it wasn't as bad as she had seen. She suggested we see what would happen if first I tried diet and exercise. I was very relieved, as I wasn't quite ready for shots and I sure did not like hospitals, so I was glad I didn't have to do an overnight stay or even check-in at all. At the clinic that day and for several days, I got a crash course in food, which was actually a gentle way to ease my personal way into diabetes. I had essentially been eating really healthfully my entire life, since my mom was a nutritionist and we hardly had any junk food or soda or even very much sugary stuff in the house. This was mostly because my mom provided veggies and salads and prepared low fat and low sugar foods. She was ahead (or maybe behind) the times. It just worked out that my dad benefited from this way of eating too. An important side note: I am extremely grateful to my mom for her forward-thinking food habits. I love all vegetables and I prefer simple, healthy food. Thanks mom!

After about a month of eating and exercising every day, my blood sugars had not normalized. My pediatrician and I agreed – I had type 1 diabetes; it was time for insulin. I knew I would feel better as soon as I started taking insulin, at least I sure hoped so, since I was feeling pretty badly all the time: tired, worn out, still thirsty. They got out an orange and some little tiny needles and a vial of saline as an insulin substitute, and I practiced a long time on that orange before I could inject myself. I still remember being surprised at how easy it was once I got the hang of it. I was also especially thankful I didn't have to go to the hospital at all. This was in part because I lived so close to the clinic and I could go in every few days. Also, since my dad had diabetes, my family knew what to do. In fact, in a weird way, I knew what to do.

One of the first things I did was go to the American Diabetes Association office in Minnesota, since we lived in St. Paul. I went by myself and when I got there, I asked to read everything they had about diabetes and how to take care of yourself. I found out I could go to "Camp Needlepoint" and, because I was sixteen, I could be a counselor-in-training. I did that for three summers and became good friends with the camp director, Alex Acker, who had diabetes, too, and was a wonderful role model of how to live with diabetes and have a great life. She understood, too, what it was like to have a family member who also had diabetes, so we shared our stories. To this day, I think having been a counselor at Camp Needlepoint was a major factor why I chose to become a high school teacher after college.

I also found out about the International Diabetes Center, the IDC, which is in St. Louis Park, Minnesota. They offered an intensive week-long diabetes training course. My dad had gone through it a few years previous to my diagnosis and he had learned lots, so I asked if I could do it too. My mom and I went and it was such an awesome week. Marion Franz was the dietitian at the IDC and she helped me learn so much about food and insulin. From day one of having type 1, I knew the secret weapon was to know as much about diabetes as I could, so I could take care of myself and live a long and awesome life.

Because of how my dad and mom treated my dad's diabetes, my diabetes was never even remotely an obstacle in my life plans. When I was a senior in high school, I went to Mexico on a school trip with the Spanish Club. I remember, one of the first things I learned to say in Spanish in high school was, *"Tengo diabetes. Por favor, no quiero comer azucar."* The translation is "I have diabetes. Please, I don't want to eat sugar." Diabetes was just something I managed in Mexico, just like I would have managed it in Minnesota. I traveled for six weeks in college in war-torn Nicaragua, Guatemala and again in Mexico. When I was a sophomore in college, I did a semester in Bogota, Colombia, and another one in Mexico City. I learned about all the shamanic cures available in Latin America for diabetes; when I told people in Mexico, in particular, that I had diabetes, they all wanted to help me. That was a really cool thing about the Mexican culture that I really liked. Unfortunately, so far, none of the offered cures have worked to cure me.

I majored in Spanish, Latin American Studies and Secondary Education. I was passionate about making the injustices of the world better and I wanted to influence young people to have open hearts and open minds. What better way to do that then to teach high school Spanish! I moved to California and got my first job at a high school in Santa Cruz. I was twenty-three years old and out on my own! As it had done for seven years, diabetes moved with me.

It's hard to know if my attention to my health influenced my general "take control" attitude, or if I was already that way and it worked out that managing my diabetes just fit in to how I approached life. In any case, I quickly became a club advisor, the leadership advisor, the student government advisor and I went to graduate school to get my administrative credential. At age twenty-nine, I became a high school administrator. That first year, I had a very stressful day one day, and I had such a bad low blood sugar reaction, that my secretary called in the school nurse, who called the paramedics. They were extremely aggressive; I was wearing a white blouse and a skirt and they jabbed the needle in my arm so roughly that a geyser of blood went all over my office and my clothes. I was completely traumatized.

They demanded that I go to the hospital in the ambulance, even though I never passed out, was not convulsing and I was completely coherent, just shaken up. In addition, they had pumped enough dextrose into me to fuel someone on a multiday endurance bike ride. I went with them to the hospital and I spent about three hours sitting in one of their beds, vowing the entire time that I would never again end up in the hospital because of diabetes, if I could help it. They released me and what I remember is that it took me several days to get my blood sugars back to normal and to regain my energy.

Shortly after this experience, which happened when I was thirty-one years old, I went to the endocrinologist and she told me my A1C was 12 percent. She told me in no uncertain terms that I was on a fast track to death. She was exceptionally brutal in her delivery of the message. I went home in tears. I was also extremely angry. I decided that thirty-one years old was too young to die and that it was time to take my diabetes management to the next level. Step One: fire that endocrinologist and hire one who would support me in my quest for wellness. Step Two: apply everything, and I mean EVERYTHING, about goal setting and project management that I had been teaching in my leadership classes to my own health.

My body and my health became my project. I did visioning, I created my mission statement, I set goals, I strategized about my resources and I made an action plan. Step Three: I hired my first personal trainer. Part of hiring her included finding out her willingness to learn about diabetes and to listen to my fears, as I navigated my way to fitness. Sue Moen was that first trainer and she sat with me as I figured out what was low blood pressure, what was low blood sugar, what was intensity and what was exertion. And through it all, she kept seeing my inner athlete and she kept believing in me.

When I was thirty-five years old, I met an endurance cyclist who had become paralyzed from the waist down in a snowboarding accident during a cliff jump. When I met Chris Klebl he wasn't yet a world medalist Paralympic Cross Country Sit-skier, but he was a competitive hand cyclist. Chris got me out on my bike and he encouraged me to go for it and enroll in a women's cycling racing clinic. When I started doing endurance cycling, my entire relationship with diabetes shifted. It was as if, one day, I was struggling with how to manage diabetes and the next day, I had motivation to figure it out. Athletics changed everything! Hanging around with paralyzed athletes who took exquisite care of themselves and who had coaches, massage therapists, and nutritionists, made me realize that people with diabetes, in this case, me, needed this too. Thus, I began my quest in earnest to assemble the best team to support me and my new goal: to ride in a 100-mile bike ride.

It took me a few years, and a move from California to Colorado, to be ready for that 100-mile ride. I did it in Moab, Utah, in the fall of 2003. At that point, I was a school development consultant and coach for Big Picture Learning, assisting high school leaders to implement the innovative Big Picture school design in their local context. This meant I traveled quite a bit, and thus had to plan my workouts in advance and take into consideration my schedule. I had found Cycling Coach, Nicole Freedman, and endocrinologist, Matt Corcoran, MD, to support me in my goal to successfully ride 100 miles in one day on my bike. The ride was epic. It took me eight and a half hours of actual riding and nine hours from start to finish, which included only thirty minutes of stopping to eat, go to the bathroom and stretch. I was very pleased, as the route was difficult and finishing was my only goal! My blood sugars remained stable and I felt on top of the world! I knew I was on to something. So much so, that I signed up in January, 2004, to ride 400 miles across the state of Colorado in the Bicycle Tour of Colorado for the summer of 2004. I trained, learned more about diabetes and exercise, and was very excited when, just a few weeks after I purchased my very first LIVESTRONG yellow bracelet, I successfully rode every mile of the Tour of Colorado! Each night on the ride, I talked to Dr. Matt and Coach Nicole. Their support and in-the-moment-coaching was invaluable.

It wasn't until after the ride was completed that things didn't go well. I just couldn't seem to recover. And my A1C skyrocketed up to 9.3 percent. Then, a week later, at a different lab, my A1C was 9.4 percent; then 8.9 percent. It made no sense. My meter wasn't correlating to these high A1C numbers. I was eating well. I had just done the most epic athletic event of my life. Dr. Matt ordered countless tests to try to figure it out. During July and August of 2004, I think I gave a gallon of blood in an effort to figure it out.

Then, in October, I was on a consulting trip for work. In my hotel room, I was doing acupressure on myself to calm my nervous system and I found a lump in my breast. Within a few days, I got the dreaded and completely unexpected diagnosis: *breast cancer*. What followed was one of the most complicated, intense trips to hell and back. For a month, all I did was have scans and tests involving lots of radioactive dye. It's a different experience than finding out about diabetes. The oncology world is amped up more than the endocrinology world. Sometimes, people die very quickly from cancer. Thus, the energy is exponentially more urgent, more dramatic. They have teams of people who make sure the patient gets scheduled to the right test, the right doctor, the right place.

In addition, people responded more intensely to hearing about cancer than they ever did to my having diabetes. Starting about five days after I found out I had breast cancer, I received a card or gift in the mail every single day for almost four solid months. It almost started to get creepy. I began to wonder if I was going to die. I never thought I would die from cancer, but the reaction of the world did catch me off guard. I found it comforting, too, and it was a little like a preview of what my funeral might be like, which was strangely cool.

Every cancer treatment regimen, just like diabetes, is unique within the overall diagnosis of cancer. I had a lumpectomy, chemotherapy and radiation therapy. Doing all of these with diabetes was particularly challenging. Each treatment component caused various interactions with my diabetes, which we had to figure out how to navigate. Every single step of the way, I had a team of support. We kept a binder of protocols, my reactions to things, and questions we had for the medical team. One particularly harrowing moment was during my first chemotherapy treatment, when we did not get the anti-nausea medications right and I ended up throwing up continuously for over twelve hours. It was absolutely the worst nightmare I had ever endured. A few profound lessons emerged from this experience. Number one: no endurance event could ever compare. Through every single race or event in which I participate, I smile and know that endurance athletes, even while suffering, enjoy a joyous thing in comparison to what else I have endured. Profound lesson number two: while I was lying on the floor for the first eight hours, before I finally agreed to go to the hospital, I felt so alone in the world with my sickness and pain. At some point, I realized that I wasn't really alone and that the feeling of aloneness wasn't my actual reality. My dearest friend was with me and so many people – my amazing family and friends – that none of us are alone. *We just THINK we are alone.* It was a spiritual awakening for me.

I finally finished chemotherapy, and the thirty-six daily rounds of radiation therapy in mid July 2005. It was a miserable year, but I made it. Well, almost. At that point, I was more physically spent than I had ever been. A strange and somewhat unusual side effect occurred: I had a concentration disorder. I was unable to focus on anything for longer than about five minutes. Since I relied heavily on my ability to focus for nearly everything in my life, my medical team convinced me that I needed some time off to heal from the ordeal I had just been through. Besides, I still had diabetes and I needed to re-focus on my diabetes management.

Shortly after treatments ended, and I was recovering from my cognitive dysfunction, I started doing cancer-related events. I remember going to a concert to raise money for cancer research and, as the event got started, they asked all of us who were survivors to please stand and be recognized. I stood up and, as I stood, the tears flooded out of me. The clapping for those of us standing was so full of love and appreciation, and to have the world see my courage moved my heart. I felt some of the awfulness of what I had endured melt away.

I also started walking at Komen events and running and cycling at LIVESTRONG events. I was given pink survivor t-shirts and yellow roses as I crossed the finish lines. I did a few triathlons for cancer awareness and the race organizers had the cancer survivors start in the first or second wave, after the elite athletes. We were given special shirts to wear that said "Team Survivor." I was surprised at how much the extra cheering boosted my self-image and continued to heal me emotionally from the ordeal of cancer.

Then, I did another Tour de Cure, the bike ride for the American Diabetes Association, my beloved organization. Much to my utter dismay, there was nothing for the cyclists with diabetes. It was August, 2006, and nothing. I kept asking everyone, "Do you have diabetes?" I couldn't find my people. I got done with that ride and I sat at the ride headquarters thinking about my disappointment. And, just like every other pivotal moment of my life, I realized I had a choice: I could complain, feel sorry for myself and wish that things would change, OR, I could take action. It really is a choice how we react to things.

My action was to join the organizing committee of the Tour de Cure Colorado. I knew that part of the reason the cancer community was so patient-centered and empowered is because survivors of cancer "wake up" to an appreciation of life and many of them get involved with cancer activism. They are the ones who've made pink ribbons so prevalent. And they don't feel sorry for themselves. No – they evoke empathy and empowerment in themselves and others.

That's what I wanted to bring to the world of diabetes. During the fall of 2006 and spring of 2007, the Red Rider Recognition Program was born. Marcey Robinson, CDE, was my diabetes educator at that point. Matt had moved east and, for the cancer experience, I needed a local diabetes team; Marcey was the amazing gal I found. Marcey, and my best friend Sandria and I, raised the funds for that first Red Rider jersey, Red Rider water bottles and t-shirts. Sandria became the Finish Line announcer, as I wanted every rider with diabetes to know how appreciated, seen and celebrated they were. I also wanted everyone out riding to yell, GO RED RIDER, every time they saw one of us in the jersey, which proclaimed on the back, "I Ride with Diabetes!" The exclamation point was intentional. It meant love and joy and pride. It was the spirit of reclaiming your health by taking action to get on the bike and exercise.

211

That first year in Colorado, my goal was to have one hundred cyclists with diabetes be Red Riders. We ended up with one hundred and eleven. This past summer, five years from when we started the program, there were about 5,000 cyclists who wore the jersey proudly in over eighty-three Tour de Cure rides in forty states! The American Diabetes Association whole-heartedly embraced the program, and expanded it to the walks for diabetes. Walkers with diabetes are called Red Striders! I now travel around the country giving keynote speeches at Tour and Expo events. Earlier in my career, I had done freshman orientation keynote speeches. This experience doing public speaking continues to come in handy as I talk to audiences about Tour de Cure, having diabetes and celebrating wellness by being an athlete.

A few years into the implementation of the Red Riders, I realized that actually figuring out diabetes and being an endurance athlete was complicated. I had figured it out because I assembled a team. Dr. Matt, Coach Nicole, CDE Marcey, Mental Skills Coach Carrie. I have a gift for assembling the right people in the room and getting them to talk to one another and to simultaneously help me out. I decided I needed to share my team with others. I like sharing! Thus, "Team WILD" was born – *W*omen *I*nspiring *L*ife with *D*iabetes. For the first three years, Team WILD was just for women with diabetes who wanted to do endurance athletics. The first year, Team WILD had twenty women, who trained with coaches and medical professionals to compete in the 70.3-mile half Ironman Distance Triathlon. We competed in the Austin, Texas, event. It was incredible! All of us finished and all of us did it with smiles! The seven and a half hours it took me to complete the event was amazing. I loved being in my body so powerfully! I loved the uniforms and the spirit of being on a team of women who were taking control of their health and lives through athletics. It was an incredible dream come true to see woman after woman cross that finish line!

Then, in June of 2010, I went in for a routine A1C test and it was elevated – up to 8.3 percent. I was surprised. I was a little more tired than usual. I had done my first marathon, the Big Sur Marathon, one of the harder ones in the United States, in April, and we had Camp WILD in early June, and I was traveling for my consulting work, so I wasn't worried about being tired, since it made sense. However, when I got that high A1C, I was a little spooked. So, I moved up my annual mammogram by a few weeks. It came back all clear, so I breathed and relaxed, a little bit.

In mid-July 2010, I found a lump, again. In the same breast as the first time, just in a different location, which is sort of funny, since it's not like I am a large chested woman by any stretch of the imagination! I went in right away and sure enough, breast cancer 2.0. This time, I stayed exponentially calmer. I knew the drill. I knew other cancer survivors and counted them as some of my closest friends. Cancer was still scary, but it wasn't devastating in the same way. The learning curve wasn't nearly so steep. And I did my research. There was no official scientifically-proven correlation between my high A1C and the fact that I had an active breast cancer tumor. However, in my case, it happened both times. In general, there IS scientific evidence that cancer grows more quickly in the presence of elevated glucose. Over the years, my oncologist often referred to me as her most highly educated patient. I took the research component of my health very seriously. I believed that to be empowered, one must have information. And do something with that information, namely the higher order thinking of Bloom's taxonomy: analysis, synthesis and evaluation. I'm the one whose body is growing cancer, and who has diabetes, thus it is my responsibility to acquire knowledge and then use the knowledge to guide my life.

Treatment for cancer 2.0 was a mastectomy. I am something of a minimalist, so I chose a unilateral. For the surgery, I approached it in the most spiritual, Zen, empowered manner possible. I crafted seven healing mantras. I love Hawaii, so I asked everyone to wear Hawaiian shirts the day of the surgery and at precisely 7:30 AM to recite the seven mantras for me, wherever they were. That was the moment surgery started. I scheduled an acupuncture treatment in pre-op for twenty-five minutes prior to going into surgery. I arranged for this with the Complimentary Medicine Center that was located in the hospital where I had the surgery. I had received acupuncture regularly for over twenty-five years, so I was not suddenly doing something new on race day, which any athlete would tell you is a no-no.

The other thing that was awesome was that I convinced the surgeon and the hospital to allow Stacy, a diabetes educator/nurse, in the operating room to monitor my diabetes. Typically the anesthesiologist is in charge of diabetes, and very few of them are specifically trained for that. This was not something I was willing to leave up to random chance. Stacy, Marcey and I worked over several weeks to plan my diabetes/insulin strategy on surgery day. I had a written plan that I shared with everyone. It was very clear and simple. I went into surgery with a blood sugar of 180 mg/dL and came out at 130 mg/dL. It was smooth and, as a result, I felt and looked amazing when it was over. My recovery was quite speedy. I started physical therapy five days after surgery and I started an easy exercise regimen one day after. I wasn't aggressive, but I was active. The body prefers movement as part of healing and I wanted to help my body as much as I could!

During the weeks after diagnosis, and then after the surgery, and during recovery while more tests were done, I had the opportunity to ask my "Inner MD", what's up? Why did I get cancer a second time? (This concept of "Inner MD" is explained by cancer activist and wellness revolutionary Kris Carr.)

213

Here's what I discovered: clearly, I have a sensitive system. Thus, I need to respond on several levels. Immediately upon diagnosis, I started some deep research about nutrition. I already ate well, but could I do better? It turned out yes, I could eat better. With the information I had gathered, I made some drastic dietary changes. It's called the "Mari diet." It resembles a vegan diet. I eat mostly organic plants. Lots of fruits and veggies. No meat. No chicken. Almost no fish. No dairy products. That means, no butter, no milk, no cheese. I eat very little sugar. And very little processed food of any sort. I only drink alcohol a few times a year. I want to protect my liver so it can process estrogen appropriately. I eat eggs, but only if they are organic and cage free. I spend a lot of time and money on food. And I will do this for the rest of my life, with a smile and joy in my heart. I call *Whole Foods* my "wellness pharmacy."

In addition to my radical shift in diet, my overall goal is to reduce inflammation in my body. So I meditate daily for at least five minutes. This reminds my system of calm and focus. I also remind myself to breathe fully about 500 times a day. Anytime I think of it, I say to myself "Breathe." Cancer grows in the absence of oxygen, so I want as much oxygen in my system as possible.

I also realized that cancer 2.0 was an opportunity to re-focus my daily reality. I want to share who I am and what I have discovered and what I have created to support people through health obstacles and challenges. Puking on the floor, having people wear Hawaiian shirts, eating mostly plants, all this brought into clear, sharp focus that we each only get one life in one body at a time, so we better wake up and listen to what our deepest purpose is. Mine is to share how the mindset of being an athlete changes everything. Athletes, high caliber athletes in particular, have a team to help them. Athletes think about nutrition, exercise, stress, sleep, medication from the lens of performance. Athletes handle set backs with grace and strategy. Endurance athletes see and experience time in cycles.

With this second cancer came the insight that I am only one person, and I had better put my energy and time toward my purpose. Sharing how our most powerful gifts emerge out of our deepest pain and vulnerability is what I am uniquely positioned to model. Thus, I am moving in the direction of making Team WILD, which is now co-ed, and stands for *We Inspire Life with Diabetes*, my full-time work. We are in collaboration with the American Diabetes Association and other wonderful and powerful organizations. I can hardly wait to discover what and how my life will continue to unfold. What I know for certain is that I am not alone and that I am, like each of us is, deeply loved and that we each have something to offer. I am grateful to all of the health challenges I have been given this lifetime. It's just another way to have a really big life adventure. GO WILD!

Website: www.teamwild.org

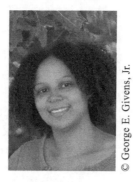

© George E. Givens, Jr.

Chapter 21 *by Cherise Shockley*

HUMANS with a Bad Pancreas

I had a normal life growing up. My mother, Nina Howard, raised me along with my five brothers. She was strict. I was the only girl; a tomboy for my entire life. I enjoyed eating Halloween candy, getting my belly full on Thanksgiving Day, and eating ice cream and cake. I do not remember anyone from my family discussing diabetes or checking their blood sugar. I was always told everything happens for a reason. The older I get, I believe it. The longer I live with diabetes, I believe it even more.

Adulthood

In the summer of 2002, I went to annual training with my Army Reserve Unit; I was in a transportation unit, but I was the Unit Supply Specialist. Our mission was to help an active duty unit transport trucks from Beaumont, Texas, to Fort Polk, Louisiana. I was excited about it! We had a real mission. On our way from Kansas City, Missouri, to Beaumont, Texas, I developed a crush on a Staff Sergeant. He seemed out of my league. I was a specialist and he out-ranked me. He was arrogant and way too confident for me. But there was something about him. When I didn't see him, I would go out of my way to look for him. I was scared. I had never felt this way about any man, especially one in uniform. I always said I would never date anyone wearing a uniform, but there was *something* about him. We arrived in Beaumont, Texas, and the training began. My supervisor wanted me to drive to Fort Polk to order and exchange uniforms. I was upset and refused to go alone. Staff Sergeant Scott Shockley volunteered to go on the trip with me.

The ride was relaxing; we had a chance to talk about life and each other. I was a little nervous. I still could not figure out why I was attracted to him. When we arrived at our destination, we jumped out of the truck. He grabbed my hand and he kissed me. After that, we were inseparable. I moved in with him a week later. We were engaged three months later and married one year after our engagement. He was deployed to Iraq two months after we said, "I do."

"You have Diabetes!"

I received a call from my mother-in-law, Judy, who told me that there was a family emergency. Scott's grandmother had passed away. I contacted the Red Cross; they filtered the message to Scott's chain of command. A few days later, Scott was on his way home. Unfortunately, he didn't make it home in time for the funeral. But I was glad to see him! We were newlyweds and "Uncle Sam" snatched Scott away before we could celebrate being married. We couldn't go on a honeymoon. So, we decided to hangout. A few days before Scott had to return to Iraq, I had a yeast infection. (What an inconvenient time for a yeast infection to interrupt my life!) I tried "over-the-counter" medications, but nothing helped. I drove Scott to the airport and an hour later he boarded the plane.

I knew something wasn't right. I called the Military Treatment Facility to schedule an appointment.

"Hi, my name is Cherise Shockley. I have an appointment with the nurse practitioner."

The woman behind the counter asked for my military ID. I gave her the card and she asked me to have a seat in the waiting area. A few minutes later, a nurse walked into the room. She asked if I was pregnant. I let her know I wasn't. She asked, "The reason for this appointment is for a yeast infection?"

I replied, "Yes, I have had a yeast infection for a few days and it will not go away. I tried over the counter medication, it did not help."

The nurse asked, "Have you lost any weight?"

I replied, "Yes, I have lost about ten pounds in the past few weeks. I've also had to use the bathroom a lot, and drinking a lot of sugary drinks and water."

The nurse led me into the exam room. I heard a knock at the door and the nurse practitioner entered the room. She asked me a few questions. I explained that I lost ten pounds, I go to the bathroom in the middle of the night, and I have a terrible yeast infection.

She asked, "Do you have a family of history of diabetes?"

I responded, "NO!"

She said, "I want to test your blood glucose levels." She pulled out a meter, pricked my finger and the meter read 334 mg/dL. She looked at me and said, "You have diabetes!" I asked her to repeat herself. Then, I cried. She held me in her arms. She said I would be okay. I was sad because I had diabetes, but felt even worse because my husband was in Iraq. She gave me a blood glucose meter and started me on *metformin* (an oral medication). She wanted me to come back the next day to have blood drawn for the labs.

I called my mom. "Mom, I have diabetes." My mom was quiet for a moment. Then she said she should have known I had diabetes because of all of the fluid I had been drinking and the frequent trips to the bathroom I was making. She said she didn't know anyone in our family who had diabetes. After I hung up the phone, I cried a little more. I called my uncle, on my dad's side, to see if there was anyone on my father's side of the family who had diabetes. My uncle said we did not have a family history of diabetes, type 1 or type 2. I knew my life would be different – but I didn't know how different it would be.

A few days later, I returned to the Military Treatment Facility to find out the results from my blood work. I walked into the room where the nurse practitioner was already seated. She looked a little perplexed. I sat down next to her. She told me that my A1C was 14.5 percent. She paused. She said, "You have the antibodies like a person living with type 1 diabetes, but your pancreas is still working like someone living with type 2 diabetes. I'm confused. I want to send you to an endocrinologist. I want you to keep taking the *metformin*, since it's helping."

I sat in disbelief. "What is going on with my body? Do I really have diabetes?"

A few weeks later I had my first appointment with the endocrinologist. After we did our meet and greet, he said, "I'm pretty sure you have type 1.5 – also known as LADA, or *Latent Autoimmune Diabetes in Adults*."

I asked, "What is Type 1.5?"

He said, "It's the slow onset of type 1 diabetes." He said he wanted me to go to the lab to have more blood work done because he didn't want to misdiagnose me. I went to the lab to have thirteen viles of blood drawn!

A week later, I had another visit with the endocrinologist. He confirmed his original hypothesis, "You have type 1.5 / LADA."

I was speechless. I knew very little about type 1 and type 2, but I had never heard of type 1.5/LADA! He said, "A lot of adults are misdiagnosed with type 2, when they have type 1.5/LADA. Your pancreas is still working, but the antibodies will attack your pancreas. You can continue to take oral medication to treat your diabetes. I need you to know that one day your pancreas will stop working and you will need insulin."

I asked, "When will I need insulin? Will I have to take shots?"
He said, "I'm not sure when your pancreas will stop working; it could be today, tomorrow or four years down the road. I am not sure. Yes, you will have to take insulin injections or use an insulin pump."

"I want to stay on oral medication and, when I need to, then I'll switch to insulin." I left the endocrinologist a little overwhelmed and confused. I knew I would be okay, but I didn't know what to expect.

New Beginnings

I joined the gym, counted carbohydrates, and took my medicine every single day. I maintained an A1C under 7.0 percent. I felt good. My husband was due home any day. I wondered what he would think. I had lost a lot of weight and ate a little differently. In March of 2005, Scott returned home from Iraq. I was excited to see Scott; it had been almost a year. I wondered what he was going to do when he saw me check my blood sugar for the first time or count my carbohydrates.

Scott walked off the bus and we ran to each other and embraced. It was a great moment in my life. Diabetes took a back seat.

In April 2005, I found out that Scott and I would be expecting our first child. I was excited and nervous. I was on oral medication; I didn't know how my life would be with diabetes and carrying a child. I immediately called my nurse practitioner. She referred me to an obstetrician-gynecologist. I also called my endocrinologist. I was told to stop taking the oral medication and I would have to start taking insulin injections. My obstetrician-gynecologist decided he wanted to be in charge of my overall diabetes care. I went home from my appointment with a bottle of insulin and a few syringes. I told Scott that I had to give myself an injection. He asked if I needed help and I told him no. I stood in the bedroom with my shirt pulled up and the insulin drawn in the syringe. I looked at myself and looked down at my stomach. I told myself that I could do it. A few minutes later, I was still standing in the same spot looking in the mirror, telling myself I can do it. But, I couldn't. I was afraid to give myself a shot in the stomach. I never had to stick a needle in anything, let alone myself. I didn't want to hurt the unborn baby that I was carrying. I called Scott into the room. I told him I was scared. He wrapped his hand around my hand. I said, "On the count of five, we are going to inject the insulin."

"1-2-3-4, I can't do it. I can't do it. Scott, I'm scared. I can't do it!"
Scott calmly replied, "Yes, you can."
I said, "Let's try it again. 1-2-3." I paused. "Scott, I can't! I'm too scared!"

Ten minutes later, Scott and I were still standing in front of the mirror holding a syringe full of insulin. I was freaking out; he was very calm.

Scott said, "Cherise, I'm going to count to five. Then *I* will insert the needle." I closed my eyes. Scott counted to five and injected the insulin into my stomach. I survived my first insulin injection with the help of my husband! I wished I had had an orange to practice on, instead of a belly with a baby inside it.

Throughout my pregnancy, I was carefully monitored. I was also a little worried because I had read a lot of stories about women living with diabetes having large babies. Scott would always tell me not to worry, but during my pregnancy, that was easier said than done. During the first trimester, I visited my obstetrician every two weeks. One day, I finally stopped blaming myself and hating my diabetes. Then I started to enjoy being pregnant. I enjoyed the little girl that was growing inside of me. The pregnancy went well. Scott and I delivered our little girl, via Caesarean section, on November 29, 2005. She weighed 6 pounds 2 ounces.

Diabetes Burnout

A few weeks after giving birth to my daughter, the endocrinologist had to make changes to my oral medications. He added *glipizide* to the *metformin* that I was taking. He also diagnosed me with *hypothyroid*. At the same time, Scott received orders to move to Southern California. I hated to leave my endocrinologist in Kansas City. I was given the okay by my endocrinologist to see an internal medicine doctor for everything related to diabetes.

It was a little over two years since I had been diagnosed with diabetes. I got tired of counting carbohydrates, exercising, and testing my blood sugar. I was mentally and physically burned out from the everyday wear and tear of the diabetes routine. Scott was very supportive, but he really couldn't understand how I felt because he doesn't have diabetes. I pretty much said "forget it"; I took my medicine and that's about all I did.

My mother-in-law came to visit during Christmas. She asked me how I was doing. I would respond with, "I am fine." Then, I decided to check my blood sugar, after eating a low carbohydrate meal. The meter read 218 mg/dL. I paused. 218 mg/dL?!?! This could not be right. I waited a few hours and tested my blood glucose levels again. The meter read 200 mg/dL. I was in a panic. The first thought that came to my mind was "my pancreas is not working." I called my Nurse Practitioner to tell her what was going on and she told me I needed to take more *metformin*. I tried explaining that I had type 1.5/LADA, not type 2. I needed to see an endocrinologist. I tried taking more *metformin*; it did not work to bring my blood sugars under control. She finally realized that she could not help me any longer because she couldn't figure out what was going on. She referred me to an endocrinologist.

Bum Pancreas

At my first visit to the new endocrinologist, I decided to see the nurse practitioner. I had visited a lot of nurse practitioners in the past, I figured why not see another one? I walked into the room, sat down, and immediately explained everything that was going on with me. I also explained the whole type 1.5/ LADA to him. I was thankful he already knew what it was. He said it seemed like the "honeymoon phase" was over and I may need to start taking insulin. Honestly, I knew he was going to say that, but I don't think it really registered. I knew, three years ago, that I would someday become insulin dependent, but I wasn't ready for it. I don't think that any child, parent of a child living with diabetes, or an adult living with diabetes, can truly say they are ready for insulin therapy. My nurse practitioner started me out on long acting insulin and four to six shots of fast acting insulin (before meals) per day. We discussed using an insulin pump versus multiple daily injections, insulin to carbohydrate ratios, carrying glucose tablets, and the list goes on and on. I left the appointment feeling overwhelmed. I called Scott to tell him I had to be on insulin for the rest of my life. I cried with him on the phone. He told me everything would be okay and I believed him. I blamed myself for a moment. What did I do wrong? Why did I have diabetes? But, then I stopped myself. I prayed and asked God to hold my hand. I left diabetes at the altar. God would never give me more than I could bear.

A few days later, I returned to visit my nurse practitioner. We discussed more about insulin pumps versus multiple daily injections. I finally decided to go on pump therapy. This time I didn't walk out of the office crying. I left with a smile on my face. I thanked God. I called my mom. I knew I had a lot of research to do.

I'm not Alone

I logged on to the Internet to see if there were any reviews about the insulin pump I decided to use. I put in the pump information into the Google search engine. I could not believe what I found. I found TuDiabetes.org. I browsed around the online diabetes community to see what type of reviews they had about my future insulin pump. I was excited. I decided to dig a little deeper and read more about this online community I found. I read blogs, message boards and recipes all from people living with diabetes and parents of children who live with diabetes. I was amazed. I decided to join TuDiabetes.org. I entered my profile. I didn't think they would have type 1.5/LADA listed under the registration but they did. I closed my eyes and screamed "I finally found a place to call home!" I called Scott to tell him the good news (he was away). He was happy for me and glad I found a place to share my thoughts and get feedback from other people living with diabetes. I couldn't stay away from <u>TuDiabetes. org</u>. If I wasn't at work or taking care of my family, I was participating in forum discussions on <u>TuDiabetes.org</u> or reading what everyone had to say about their lives with diabetes. I made sure I asked questions about being on an insulin pump, using insulin, carbohydrates and transitioning from oral medication to insulin. I received a lot of great responses from people in the community. I was comfortable with this community of strangers; they understood what life is like with diabetes. I didn't feel like I was the only person living with diabetes. I realized I wasn't alone.

Telling my Story

I was plugged into to the Diabetes Online Community (DOC). I read a lot of amazing blogs from people living with type 1 diabetes, there were a few blogs about people with type 2 diabetes, but there were even fewer blogs written by people with type 1.5/LADA. I decided to create my own blog to document my life with diabetes. I needed a way to talk about the good times with diabetes and vent my feelings about the bad times. I wanted to share my story in hopes of helping someone else. I called my mother and we went over a few choices for my blog name. I wanted a name that meant something personal to me. My mother and I came up with "Diabetic_Iz_Me" (please see my Website list at the end of this chapter). I called Scott to see what he thought. He really liked it. I was a little nervous about sharing my personal journey with diabetes on the Internet, but my heart told me I needed to do it. I prayed about it. Then, I put my fingers on the keyboard and I'm glad I did.

Diabetes and People Living with It Inspire Me

I gained a whole new outlook on living with diabetes and what others go through by reading blogs, using Twitter, and participating in communities such as TuDiabetes.org. The DOC is a large community with a HUGE heart, full of inspiration, support, determination and willpower to not let diabetes win. The DOC inspires me.

I refuse to let diabetes kill my spirit or steal my joy; some days are better than others. Diabetes can be a frustrating disease; every day is different. I am not going to lie – sometimes I want to throw the stupid meter across the room, give up, and cry. But, I won't let it win. People living with diabetes are more than just a number: we are wives, mothers, husbands, brothers, sisters and friends. We are HUMANS with a bad pancreas!

I can't hate something I have to live with for the rest of my life. I have to live with it. I do not suffer from diabetes. I have diabetes. I live with it. I leave the negative thoughts, out of range numbers and the bad feelings I have about diabetes, at the altar. I have learned to embrace and manage diabetes. I am thankful for all of the positive things diabetes has brought into my life. I am blessed to have the friendships and extended family. I'm empowered, inspired and motivated by diabetes. I am a stronger person because of it.

Website: www.diabetic-iz-me.com

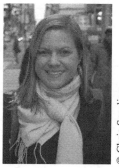
© Chris Sparling

Chapter 22 *by Kerri Morrone Sparling*

A Shifting Definition of Success

I liked to climb trees. It was a hobby of mine, as a seven-year-old. My brother and sister and I would play in the yard all day in the summer, building forts and riding bikes and shimmying up trees like little monkeys. The view from the base of the tree was always so amazing, looking up into the highest branches, trying to count the seemingly millions of leaves, and wondering what kind of birds made their homes up there.

"Do you think there are pterodactyls up there?" my sister asked, shielding her eyes from the sun.

"Yes," I replied, a dinosaur expert at the time, having just completed the first grade. "Giant ones. With party hats." (Okay, maybe "expert" was a stretch.)

Once I scurried up a few branches, the view changed. The world looked remarkable from that higher vantage point, with the blades of grass just far enough away that they were blurry, but the leaves were all around me and I could see ladybugs and caterpillars moving along in their buggy traffic patterns. Reaching those higher branches made me feel like I was successful, like I had done something that made me feel proud and that changed my perspective.

That summer before starting the second grade, I started to wet the bed again. Nothing too dramatic, but enough that my parents were concerned. I seemed healthy, otherwise, so their response to this odd bedwetting revival was to buy an alarm that connected to my underpants.

"If you start to urinate, these two metal pieces will connect and an alarm will go off. That way, you won't wet the bed and you can get up and use the bathroom!" My mom seemed pleased, hoping this would fix the problem.

"Okay," I said. I was embarrassed that I was wetting the bed. I hadn't wet the bed in years. I wore the bedwetting alarm for about two weeks, and after waking up almost every night with my underpants going off like a fire engine siren, I was scared straight.

I spent the rest of the summer climbing trees, sleeping over at my friends' houses, and being a kid. Never wet the bed again. But something was still a little bit off.

A few weeks before I was scheduled to start school, my mother took me in for my before-school physical.

(Never in my life had so many people been so interested in my urine.)

"Just wipe with these special wipes – front to back, Kerri – and urinate into the cup. Close it up, bring it out, and we'll have everything we need!" The nurse smiled at me while my mother and the pediatrician talked about how excited I was to start school.

I did what they asked, and a few days later, we received a call back from the pediatrician's office. My parents repeated words I didn't understand – "diabetes" and "hospital" – and the whirlwind of change began.

I was diagnosed with type 1 diabetes on September 11, 1986. I spent twelve nights in Rhode Island Hospital, learning to give practice injections of saline to an orange.

"We use an orange because its skin is most like human skin," the diabetes educator explained. Which is when it dawned on me that these needles were intended for my skin. And at that moment, success was redefined by having the guts to press these needles into my body, every day, for the rest of my life.

The weeks that followed were a flurry of doctor's appointments, hospital stays, midnight lab work appointments, food scales, and injections. The thing about type 1 diabetes is that you go from diagnosis to intense management in a matter of 24 hours. On the day before my diagnosis, I went to bed without checking my blood sugar and didn't give any thought at all to the carbohydrate content of my snack. I didn't stick a needle into my arm and inject insulin that was stolen from the pancreas of a cow. My mother didn't worry about how stable my numbers would be throughout the night. I just went to bed.

The night after my diagnosis, we were learning about our new "normal." It was like being high up in those treetops again, adjusting to the confusing new view.

Being diagnosed with type 1 diabetes at such a young age gives me a certain emotional advantage, because I do not recall much about life at all without this disease. I have fuzzy memories of going to Disney World and playing in the tree fort in our backyard, but they're all blended together, those memories. I can't remember what was "before" and what was "after." Life with diabetes has simply always been 'life' for me. It's difficult to long for that "before" when you don't remember it. But that kind of emotional advantage is often overshadowed by the physical disadvantage. Currently, I'm barely into my 30's, with twenty-five years of a serious chronic illness under my belt. Complications as a result of this many years with diabetes could be part of my youth, but I can't dwell on that. I feel like I don't have time for that, not at this point. Diabetes is part of my life, and who I am, making "acceptance without apathy" part of me, too. But it's not a choice. Diabetes just . . . is.

I don't remember growing up with diabetes as being a big inconvenience, or even part of the daily focus. School dances, summer jobs, first kisses . . . all with diabetes as part of the "me" package. Everyone in my family knew I had diabetes, and almost all of my friends were aware, so after the initial awkwardness of meeting and explaining things to new friends, I was off and running without much pause. I understood that the decisions I made would affect my future, in one way or another, but I had a good sense that as it pertained to all things, so too, diabetes wasn't an exception. Some things in life are challenging, and diabetes happens to be one of them.

However, I was the only kid I knew who had type 1 diabetes. My small Rhode Island town wasn't big enough at the time for two grocery stores, never mind a whole diabetes community, so finding other kids whose pancreases didn't produce insulin was difficult. This marked lack of community was hard, both for my parents and for me. In efforts to help me connect with other kids who really understood, my parents signed me up for Clara Barton Camp for Diabetic Girls (now known as The Barton Center), and for twelve days, I was surrounded by other little girls who also shot up before they ate breakfast. I was empowered, knowing I wasn't alone, and that there was life – a good life – to be had after diagnosis. Unfortunately, with the end of camp came the end of my access to a diabetes community. When I graduated high school in 1997, I was one of three kids with type 1 diabetes in our school district. None of my friends had diabetes, and there weren't any other people with diabetes in my family. I felt proud of my accomplishments in taking care of my health and my diabetes, but I didn't know who to "high-five," because no one else seemed to understand how proud I felt when the meter showed a nice, round "100" mg/dL. Regardless of the fact that I threw parties with my friends, went on dates, and graduated in the top of my class, there was still that desire to find others "like me," who were living with diabetes, too. I kept searching for my community.

Success, when I was a little kid with diabetes, was following my mom's careful directions and having numbers that didn't make my endocrinologist cluck her tongue against the roof of her mouth as she poured through my logbook. (Which, at times, she did. Puberty was a tough time for a young girl with diabetes – all those wildly fluctuating hormones made for a hornet's nest of blood sugar numbers.) It was about making her proud, and staying safe.

229

Diabetes wasn't the sole focus of my childhood, and I had this luxury because my mother worked so hard on my behalf. She made sure that my life was as unaffected by diabetes as possible. While I slept, she would sneak into my room at six in the morning to inject me with my morning dose of NPH. Three months after my diagnosis, I had my first sleepover at a friend's house. My mother was terrified to let me go, but knew my independence and my happiness were just as important as my health. So she brought me to my friend's house, stayed chatting with my friend's mom until it was time for my bedtime shot, and gave me my insulin injection before driving home. And the following morning, she was there again, having coffee with my friend's mom and then waking me up to give me my morning injection. She made sure I saw my endocrinologist every three months, and that I tested my blood sugar. She kept me safe. And she worried so I wouldn't have to. My mother, for those formative years as we both learned the ropes of life with type 1 diabetes, was my pancreas. But she and I knew that, as I grew up, I would need to take on full responsibility for my disease. While I looked forward to graduating high school and going away to college, my mother was nervous.

I attended college at the University of Rhode Island and made some of my closest friendships, but again, my pancreas was the only one in the bunch that was on vacation. College life for me was just like college for my seven roommates, only with a few extra hiccups. (Like when we rented a seven-room bed and breakfast as our house for Junior year, and I had to explain why the butter compartment was going to be the home for my insulin bottles instead of our butter. Or when we bought two little plastic bears filled with honey at the grocery store, marking one in black Sharpie marker as "KERRI'S!!!") I had a lot of support, though, even when my friends didn't really understand what they were supporting.

During my college years, success was defined by my grade point average and my A1C. Very proper, very quantifiable determinants. But when my parents went through a very complicated divorce, the summer between my sophomore and junior years, my world tilted a bit more on its axis, and things weren't as easy to pinpoint anymore. I was thrown into a depression with anxiety that I hadn't ever experienced before, and it redefined my perception of success. Success wasn't about being top of my class, or having an A1C that rivaled that of a person without diabetes. It wasn't about being able to check certain accomplishment boxes. At that moment in my life, when I felt disconnected from security and stability, success became defined by being happy and feeling whole.

Going through that experience with my family split us apart in some ways, but brought us together in just as many. However, it also showed me that my health is drastically affected by my emotional condition, and being psychologically unsettled makes my diabetes management a crisis. As my family recovered and rebuilt, I needed to find the same solace for my diabetes-related emotional health. But finding community was a challenge, being from a small town in the smallest state.

The themes of community and loneliness have been recurrent in my diabetes life. When I was a young child, diabetes was dealt with as a family affair. My mother planned my meals, helped me test my blood sugar, and came to every appointment with me at the Joslin Diabetes Clinic in Boston. My brother and sister had to deal with diabetes' attention-seeking ways and the fear that something would happen to their sister . . . or that they might be diagnosed with diabetes, too. My father was responsible for keeping our family financially stable so that my mother could cut her work back to part-time in order to take care of my medical needs. My diabetes was mine, but only technically. In reality, it belonged to my family as well.

But, try as they might to understand, their empathy could only go so far. Just as I had no idea what it was like to care for a child with diabetes, my parents didn't understand what it was like to be that child with diabetes. I tried to explain how a low blood sugar felt, or a high one, but my words could only resonate to a certain point. I craved understanding, kindred spirits, and their absence in my childhood left a gaping hole. I felt alone. Alone with diabetes, yet oddly still part of the diabetes community. No one knew I was there, but just hearing someone at school mention, "their cousin has type 1," or "That lady they were waiting on at the restaurant, she freaked out when her diet soda was switched – she said she had diabetes," made me feel like I was instantly connected to these imperfect strangers.

My definition of "support" changed the day I met my husband. "So what is that, an insulin pump?" He asked, and I was so taken aback that this handsome guy knew what this device was for that I responded with a flustered, "Yes?" When we first met, his perception of diabetes was vague and faceless, and the only tangible symptom I had, as far as he was concerned, was the insulin pump attached to my hip. I had to learn how to explain diabetes in a way that would educate and not scare my future husband, and he had to listen and learn to love me without fear. We began to build our future together, knowing that it involved this thing called diabetes, but that my life, and our relationship, wasn't defined by this disease.

After several months of dating, he encouraged me to share my thoughts about diabetes on a web blog. "It's a blog, like an online journal, and you can tell your story to the world through that one web page. Maybe you'll find other twenty-somethings, like you, who have had diabetes for a long time." He understood that support meant more than just sharing my feelings with him. He knew that I needed those kindred spirits whose pancreases also neglected to produce their own insulin. On a very sunny afternoon in May, after spending the day walking along the beach, I decided to start a blog. On May 4, 2005, I wrote my first blog post about life with type 1 diabetes at www.SixUntilMe.com (six years until my first symptoms of diabetes). It's funny how fast the words come when they've been bottled up inside of you for almost two decades. And from that moment on, I found my community. I knew where I belonged and I didn't feel alone anymore.

"Diabetes doesn't define me, but it helps explain me." It's the tagline of my blog, and it's become the mantra by which I manage my health. Diabetes doesn't define who I am or what I will become, but it does help explain why I wear this insulin pump, and this continuous glucose monitor. It explains why my pharmacist knows me by my first name, and why the endocrinologist sees me more often than some of my own family members. And it also explains why my family has extended to include people I haven't even met. Face-to-face interaction is such a huge part of feeling like a community, but it's not the only thing that makes us feel connected as "one." Whether you want to be part of the diabetes community or whether you are rebelling against the very thought, the fact remains that it's there for you, and will always be there for you. There's a certain comfort to knowing you aren't isolated or alone. There are people who understand.

The definition of the diabetes community is found in the people who are part of it. Each and every one of us: the bloggers, the medical professionals who care for us, the parents of kids with diabetes, the kids with diabetes who have grown up to become parents themselves, the lovers, boyfriends, girlfriends, spouses, friends of people with diabetes, the immediate family members and the ones who are slightly removed, the employers, the employees, the strangers who help us get juice when we can't help ourselves, the friends, Romans, and countrymen ARE the diabetes community.

It's a far-reaching group of people who share more than just a busted pancreas. It's a true community of people who understand, despite different backgrounds and preferences and opinions. And being part of this group brings me a sense of emotional peace when it comes to diabetes. Connecting with thousands of kindred spirits on a daily basis, and sharing our lives with diabetes in a way that empowers and educates us as a community! Being blessed enough to call my "job" and my "passion" by the same name! Feeling at peace with a disease that seems bent on making my life challenging! This, to me, is redefining success yet again.

Throughout my life, success has been a constantly-evolving concept, but I believe I've achieved true success in a goal I achieved in April of 2010. When I was diagnosed with type 1 diabetes in 1986, I was told that conceiving and carrying a child would be next-to-impossible. I believed this for many years, and after other fertility issues unrelated to diabetes, I had very little hope that I would have a child.

But through the help of my incredible medical team at the Joslin Diabetes Clinic in Boston, Massachusetts, I began my mission towards motherhood. After seeing other women with diabetes in the online community achieving their goals of becoming moms, I felt inspired and encouraged that a happy, healthy baby could be part of my future, too. My husband and I worked together to get my diabetes under the tightest control I could manage, and in August of 2009, we were humbled to find out I was pregnant.

Success, during those months of my pregnancy, was redefined during every ultrasound. I have never been so focused and so determined to keep myself as healthy as I was while pregnant. Success was waking up to a fasting blood glucose of 90 mg/dL. Success was hearing my daughter's heartbeat and seeing her little hands waving from inside the womb. Success was that morning in April of 2010, when our family expanded to embrace a wiggly little girl with a full head of hair and chubby legs. Despite a stressful pregnancy, including preeclampsia, a month of bed rest, and a Cesarean section delivery, I achieved my greatest and most life-changing goal: becoming a mom. Her mom.

It's been twenty-five years since my type 1 diabetes diagnosis, and life is still built on quicksand. You never know what the next day will bring, for better or for worse, but living with a chronic illness helps shape my perspective towards something more appreciative of the joys I do have. Being successful, to me, is feeling happy. I currently make my living as a diabetes advocate, writing about life with diabetes and helping to empower patients across the globe. Being able to stay home and raise my daughter, while working in a job that nourishes my soul, brings me a joy I didn't understand was possible. My days mean something, at least to me, and that kind of fulfillment is a blessing. I appreciate my marriage, my daughter, and the love and support of my extended family and friends. Diabetes has not stopped me from living the life I want, but instead just brings this added layer of emotional and physical complexity. I'm prepared to work hard, and to try and enjoy the ever-changing view from wherever I am.

My daughter is sixteen months old now, and she walks with her hands in the air, waving with excitement. Sometimes we sit at the bottom of the pear tree in the backyard and look up, up, up into the branches. Someday, she will understand what diabetes means. Someday, she will pave her own successful path, and her perspective will grow with every step.

"Do you see that, baby girl? Do you see?" She cranes her neck in effort to see the highest branch, the smallest leaf. And in those moments, my success is redefined by her smile.

Website: www.SixUntilMe.com

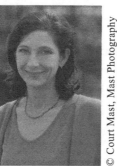
© Court Mast, Mast Photography

Chapter 23   *by Amy Tenderich, MA*

When Diabetes Alters Your Life Course, Be Sure You Grab the Wheel

Blindsided

You never know when your life will change, both suddenly and profoundly. For me, there have been two events that altered the course of my life. These events made me re-think both my priorities and the way I viewed myself as a citizen of this world; these were becoming a mother, and becoming a person with diabetes.

At the age of thirty-seven, five months after my third daughter was born, I was diagnosed with type 1 diabetes. At the time, this was a mysterious illness that had been heretofore only diagnosed in "juveniles." How could I, a fit and trim thirty-something working mother, contract diabetes? Especially the "childhood" autoimmune kind? I honestly felt like the only adult on the planet who had ever experienced this. The doctors I first encountered offered nothing in the way of support, or any help with coping.

Suddenly, leaving the house meant I had to juggle a diaper bag chock full of milk bottles and baby gear with insulin cool packs, blood glucose meter and strips, glucose tablets, appropriate snacks, plus batteries and backups for everything. I had to constantly think ahead about whether and what I'd be eating and any possible form of physical exertion ahead of me, so that I could dose insulin appropriately in order not to risk passing out.

I kept thinking, "Are you kidding me? Do people really live like this? If so, where the heck are they? And is it possible to even conceive of 'succeeding' with diabetes?"

It was this deep sense of bewilderment and isolation that prompted everything I have done in the years since – from starting one of the world's first blogs on diabetes, to growing the site into a thriving patient community, to becoming a renowned patient advocate and author, and to launching a national campaign to improve the design of devices and tools that help people everywhere live better with diabetes. Due to my advocacy, I essentially (and unwittingly) became the poster child for something called type 1.5 diabetes, also known as LADA, or *Latent Autoimmune Diabetes in Adults*.

But first things first. Allow me to share the as-yet-untold story of my diagnosis, in the hopes that some ridiculously busy moms like me will take solace in the "balls in the air" theory.

The year was 2003. I had a five-year-old, a three-year-old and a five-month-old daughter at my hip. I was working as a freelance writer covering technology in Silicon Valley, and was feeling so profoundly exhausted that I decided to give up breastfeeding my little one early (my goal had been to breastfeed her for six months). Just after I had transitioned her to the bottle, I started losing weight. In fact, my "skinny jeans" were hanging off me in a matter of weeks.

At first I was thrilled, but then things started to get weird. The exhaustion settled in to a kind of stupor: a state of sluggishness I had never experienced before. But my baby had the flu and had been waking me up around the clock, so I thought that must be why I felt like I was walking on my knees. At that time, I was also popping allergy pills like candy to offset sinus pressure I was experiencing that seemed likely to flatten my face.

Then, my vision went blurry. I called the optometrist to complain about my contact lenses that he had just ordered for me. When a replacement pair arrived, I called again: "These are just as crappy as the last pair! I can't see anything!" Meanwhile, since the birth of my youngest child, I had suffered with a raging yeast infection that wouldn't respond to any cream or pill. The itching was insanely uncomfortable.

We had a trip planned to Disneyland, and I wasn't about to give that up! So I got in the car with my three young children and our then-nanny and drove eight hours down the coast of California, squinting my eyes and squirming to stay awake all the way.

During our first day at Disneyland, I spent at least $75 on beverages alone. I could not drink enough, or go to the bathroom enough, to obtain any relief. On the second day at Disneyland, I felt like a zombie, even though I was happy to be there with my children. On the third day, my husband flew down to meet us in Southern California. He looked taken aback when he saw me changing my shirt, as my ribs poked out. He immediately told me that something was wrong. I knew he was right, because each morning I woke up skinnier than I had been the day before!

I was scared. But I still had to get my family back where they belonged. So again, I got in the car and drove all the way up the state. I had no idea that I was in danger of passing out from *diabetic ketoacidosis*!

The first night we were back home, all I wanted to do was lie down. I felt like I could sleep for a week, if only my children and clients would leave me in peace. When I got the call from the doctor, at first I wasn't surprised. I had taken a blood test earlier that day after my primary physician had said something about suspecting diabetes, and that I could "see her in the morning" about my high blood sugar. (I did *not* understand the ramifications at that point). But the on-call doctor who'd called me on the telephone that night was frantic. He insisted that I come to the emergency room right away, or risk slipping into a coma!

At my husband's insistence, I grabbed my purse and off we went. Little did I know this would become the worst week of my life. I was constantly being poked and prodded in the hospital, which was bad enough. Worse yet, I was told that I had a lifelong illness that could easily kill me if I didn't take care of it.

I cried a lot in those first weeks. I sat on the couch and cried for my children, for my husband, and for the lost beauty and power of the uncompromised health I had enjoyed for so long, but not sufficiently appreciated until it was gone. I cried because I felt fragile and "broken," and I feared for the future.

They sent me home from the hospital with a photocopy of a "sliding scale" for insulin dosing, which "guesstimated" four to six units of insulin per meal. Little did I know that I was still in my insulin "honeymoon phase," and that a half-unit could throw me into severe *hypoglycemia*. Because of this, I felt like I was having a nervous breakdown after every meal.

I was almost afraid to leave the house. I couldn't live like this! How would I ever get a handle on this thing? It truly felt like the carbohydrate counting, the constant glucose testing, the needles and the fear had taken over my life.

Leave it to my wise mother to put everything in perspective. "You've always been a master juggler," my mom told me. "Don't I always tell you you've got so many balls in the air, and you do a wonderful job keeping them all moving? Well, this is just another ball. You'll throw the diabetes into the mix and manage it along with everything else!"

This is when I realized that my mom was right. I couldn't thank her enough for this observation, because it gave me hope at a time I desperately needed some. She reminded me that diabetes doesn't have to be the focal point. It isn't necessarily *the* challenge of your life, but *another* challenge in your life, along with many others. I got up off the couch and resolved to tackle this thing, or die trying. (Hoping the last was just a figure of speech.)

Got Resolution?

One of the first things I did was contact a friend who knew someone – another woman about my age – who had type 1 diabetes. I made a cold call and asked the woman to meet me for coffee. That was the best move I ever made. The forty-five minutes I spent with this real, live, fashionable, intelligent, bubbly young career woman lifted the shroud of diabetes doom: if she could hold down a good job, a nice apartment, an aggressive fitness routine and a fiancé to boot while keeping her diabetes under control, then surely I could, too . . . right?

There must be others out there seeking connections and answers to their real-life questions about living with diabetes, I thought. I couldn't be the only one confused and frustrated by the barrage of conflicting diabetes headlines in the newspapers. So naturally, I turned to the Internet. But back then, in 2004, all I found on the Web were reams of medical journal articles, and more conflicting headlines that told me nothing about how to live and thrive with diabetes. At that time, social media had just started to take shape due to the advent of blogging software. This might be why I wasn't able to find what I needed. Or perhaps what I needed just wasn't available yet.

It was my husband who encouraged me to start a site about diabetes. "You're going to be a blogger," he said. "It's your calling!"

Huh . . . ? I thought. But he was insistent. He helped me set up the first incarnation of DiabetesMine.com, a play-on word for "it's mine – I'm stuck with it" and the notion of "a gold mine of straight talk and encouragement for people living with diabetes."

It didn't hurt that I had a university degree and a past career in journalism, plus a Master's degree in Mass Communication Research. I'd been writing professionally for years, but was elated over this opportunity to rediscover my own voice (and use grammar at my whimsy – I have a thing for exclamation points! As you may have noticed.)

I began to report, report, report – on everything from mail order medications to the lab tests I hated most, to talking with my children about diabetes – and lo and behold, people came to the site by the dozens and began to talk back to me. The interaction was amazing, because as a traditional journalist I had never had the opportunity for dialogue with my readers. I was enthralled! In the early days, I would often stay up until 2:00 AM researching posts, messaging with others I had found in online forums, and making tweaks to my site in the hopes of making it an ever-richer resource for readers.

The other thing I began to do was network, network, network. I thought, *Why not treat diabetes like my "beat" at a newspaper by attending industry events and getting to know "who's who" in the diabetes community?* For example, I was the first blogger ever to "infiltrate" the American Diabetes Association (ADA) Scientific Sessions, back in 2005.

The fact is, much of the community wasn't well-connected back then and I felt I could help by "connecting the dots" – bringing people and isolated diabetes groups together by making them aware of each other, informing them, motivating them, offering them an outlet to laugh and to vent their frustrations and learn from each other – all of the things I thought were missing for people like me – people with diabetes (or PWD, for short).

In the early phases of all of this, I woke up one morning with the most horrendous case of hives you've ever seen (a swollen eye, a patchy neck, and arms that looked like they'd suffered third-degree burns). I visited doctor after doctor, who shrugged their shoulders and said that the origin of hives was "notoriously difficult to diagnose." Most of them thought hives had been brought on by the stress I experienced over being diagnosed with diabetes, which wasn't helpful at all.

It was only through a chance encounter online that I found another patient who pointed out that celiac disease and gluten intolerance were sometimes closely associated with type 1 diabetes. After nearly a year of suffering with this itchy disfigurement, I finally had a clue. After I cut wheat out of my diet entirely, the hives disappeared and never returned (except when I made an occasional boo-boo by eating "unsafe" foods).

This, to me, was a testament to the power of patient networking. I could get real information about the aspects of diabetes that mattered to me most. Through my own site, I have learned about all sorts of things from other PWDs: the best carry cases, medical ID jewelry and logging tools; how to handle international travel; and what it feels like to wear a pump, for example.

I figured anything that I didn't know or hadn't heard of yet would probably be interesting news for other PWDs, too. That's why I began to post reviews of both products and books on diabetes. It's also why I reported on fundraising campaigns, FDA hearings and medical adhesive wipes, and on the growing community of diabetes bloggers and networking sites that cropped up all around me.

To my gratification, people responded with enthusiasm. The whole experience was tremendously empowering. I now knew that I could help offset myths about diabetes, while deflecting the crazy mainstream media headlines that either made you want to kill yourself, or kill the reporter.

In short, my new goal was to help cut through the formal mumbo-jumbo of traditional press coverage in order to bring some much-needed "straight talk" to other inquisitive patients like me. Every time I sat down to write a post – whether it was about a new development in stem cell research or a new low-carbohydrate snack – I challenged myself to answer these fundamental questions: Why should we (PWDs) care about this item/topic/news? Who's behind it, and why? What's the real impact on our day-to-day life with diabetes? How much does it cost? And so on. By adding a healthy dose of skepticism and a dash of wit, I aimed to make articles regarding diabetes topics fun to read about.

I set out to learn everything I could about my illness and how people could live with it successfully. I wanted to understand (and help others understand) the landscape and who the "movers and shakers" were – with hopes of eventually becoming one of those movers and shakers myself one day. My aim was to make life better for PWDs.

By "better," I mean:

- easy access to social support and camaraderie
- easier access to clear, insightful information about *real life* with diabetes, i.e., a layman's interpretation of all the medical and pharmaceutical mumbo-jumbo
- increased transparency from companies that serve the "diabetes market," forcing them to recognize that their customer base is made up of the people who live with this illness every day, not just the clinicians whose job it is to help push their products
- increased respect from the doctors and other healthcare professionals who treat us, rather than condescension and disdain, with the hopes of becoming a true partner with those who treat us
- design of products and tools that make sense for patients in the real world, i.e., are *comfortable* to live with and that serve a sensible purpose without overburdening the patient

An early commenter on DiabetesMine wrote to me: "You help bridge the gap between the Medical Establishment and the patients who are blindsided by this illness." That was when I knew I had succeeded, as that's what I had aimed to do from the day I got off that couch full of resolution.

Brave New (D-)World

I built a new life around my blog, a life where my illness became both my passion and my career. I slowly phased out the work I had been doing as a technology writer and threw myself into the world of diabetes reporting and diabetes advocacy, which became closely connected with the rise of health social media and so-called Health 2.0 technology (new interactive Web-based tools that let people do things for their health online).

In 2006, Eli Lilly and Company awarded me their "LillyforLife ™ Award for Diabetes Journalism." They flew me out to their Indianapolis headquarters with a handful of other recipients for an awards ceremony and a tour of their facility. It was my first look behind the scenes at one of the "all-powerful" big pharmaceutical companies, and meeting the real people there and seeing drug production in action was eye-opening; it fueled my desire to bridge the gap between these production giants and the people whose lives depend on them.

Shortly thereafter, one of the exciting opportunities that came my way was the chance to co-author a book with a leading endocrinologist from the legendary Joslin Diabetes Center in Boston, Massachusetts. Dr. Richard Jackson, a sweet, down-to-earth man who had been researching this disease and treating diabetes patients for decades, had a vision of a handbook he wanted to offer patients. As it turned out, it was the same vision I had, of a book that would (finally) give patients like me a bigger picture of our overall health management beyond just sticking our fingers all day! *For goodness' sake,* I thought, *we patients need some help out here in the real world developing a clear strategy for living well with diabetes, and avoiding the long-term damage it can cause.*

Our handbook *Know Your Numbers, Outlive Your Diabetes* (Marlowe Diabetes Library, 2007), was designed to do just that. It's an easy-to-read, highly motivational guide to the five crucial tests that everyone living with diabetes needs to have and monitor on a regular basis: hemoglobin A1C, blood pressure, lipid profile, microalbumin and a yearly eye exam. Our handbook explains what the tests mean, when and how to get them, and most importantly, it offers step-by-step recommendations for how to bring your numbers into the healthy range if they currently are not there. I like to call it the "Do-It-Yourself" guide to staying healthy with diabetes.

I was later approached by the team at "dLife," the first-ever weekly cable TV show devoted to the topic of diabetes, to be the first-ever diabetes lifestyle columnist for their Website.

As my blog DiabetesMine continued to flourish, I began working with a small health media company based in Salt Lake City called Alliance Health Networks, writing no-nonsense articles for their weekly diabetes patient newsletter. This cooperation evolved into the opportunity to be in on the ground floor of what is now one of the most successful online patient communities on the Internet: DiabeticConnect.com. It's a Facebook-like meeting place designed specifically for the needs of people with diabetes, with interactive sections for sharing Recipes, Book Reviews, Q&A and Discussions, and even an area for rating and comparing diabetes products. Where else can you go to discover other patients' real-life experiences with a certain brand of meter, insulin, or oral drug?

In the last few years, DiabeticConnect.com has grown to over 500,000 registered members, with 870 product reviews posted to date, plus an average of twenty new discussions started daily, and an average 122 responses to each discussion. Clearly, its features are meeting a need!

In order to beef up the educational content of the site, I recently published a yearlong series of tips about living with diabetes – on everything from carbohydrate counting to drug side effects to sexual dysfunction – which appear in the "Health Center" section of the site and are soon to be compiled as a downloadable e-book.

To my delight, the notion of patient empowerment has become a national and international movement. Fueled by the Health 2.0 technologies that allow us to connect and self-publish, a whole community of online patient advocates (sometimes called "ePatients") has grown up around me – hundreds of other people sharing their health challenges on the Web. We exchange treatment and insurance tips, link to each other's work and to relevant articles, hold online chats, and even manage to meet in person sometimes.

With free access to all sorts of medical information, patients like me can drive our own care for the first time in history by asking questions and demanding the latest and greatest drugs and devices. We patients can now interact with each other and complain about providers and services out in the open. We are no longer a "silent majority" totally at the mercy of doctors and pharmaceutical companies, which has ended the stranglehold of doctors and health insurance companies on information and treatment options.

As a visible part of this movement, I've become a frequent speaker at diabetes and health/social media events. These appearances include speaking at the original Health 2.0 conference series, Mayo Clinic's Transform event, the Robert Wood Johnson Foundation's Project Health Design, the Taking Care of Your Diabetes (TCOYD) series, the Diabetes Research Institute (DRI), the Behavioral Diabetes Institute in San Diego, and a number of healthcare policy events taking place in Washington, D.C. Also, when a group of activists and forward-thinking physicians launched the Journal for Participatory Medicine in 2009, I was invited to be a member of the editorial board.

Much of my notoriety has to do with something called the DiabetesMine Design Challenge, a national competition for innovation I kicked off in 2008 to foster improved design of diabetes devices. The Challenge started as a simple gripe: the design of most tools to help manage diabetes was clunky and old-school, more suited for a hospital environment than for real life. Why couldn't diabetes devices be smaller, sleeker, more comfortable to carry and cool-looking? Like, say, an iPod?

This is why, on the occasion of Apple selling its 100 millionth iPod (in 2007), I penned a tongue-in-cheek Open Letter to Apple's CEO Steve Jobs on my own blog at DiabetesMine, asking just that question. And boy, did my post hit a nerve! It was picked up all over the blogosphere and mainstream media (TechCrunch, Medscape, *Business Week*, *Forbes*, *UK Guardian*, etc.). After that, the idea for an open innovation competition was born! I was able to secure a grant from the California HealthCare Foundation's Chronic Disease Care program, and the support of world-renown design firm IDEO, to turn this contest into an annual high-profile event with $25,000 in prize money.

The DiabetesMine Design Challenge has been credited with "lighting a fire under the medical device industry" by the Chicago Tribune. Jeffrey Brewer, President and CEO of the Juvenile Diabetes Research Foundation (JDRF), recently stated: "This contest has created a great deal of buzz within the diabetes industry, really helping to push the evolution of medical devices." My contest team and I were very proud and excited about that.

As the notion of patient empowerment through online connections began to take off, Alliance Health Networks has emerged as a pioneering developer of social health communities: besides DiabeticConnect, they've launched nearly forty other networks for health conditions including sleep disorders, back pain, fibromyalgia, celiac disease, migraines, arthritis and asthma. This is why I joined Alliance Health Networks in January of 2011 as Vice President of Patient Advocacy; my day-to-day job is primarily to act as Editor-in-Chief of DiabetesMine.com and continue my ongoing advocacy efforts.

Thus, as you see, I've turned my disease into both a personal passion and a meaningful new career – one I wouldn't change for the world.

On the personal side, being a prominent patient advocate doesn't make me a "perfect PWD" by any means. Okay, being a nationally-known blogger does have its perks: I'm often able to get my hands on new diabetes technologies quickly, sometimes free of cost, for review purposes. In 2006, I was one of the first patients in the country to test the first-ever FDA-approved continuous glucose monitor (CGM). I found the Dexcom™, and later other CGM systems, useful for trend spotting but difficult to live with over time.

But even with these advantages, I struggle with ups and downs like anyone else. My "honeymoon phase" lasted about one year. (I rarely saw numbers outside the 80 mg/dL to 116 mg/dL range!) But since the honeymoon ended, I don't mind admitting that I've been in a state of semi-shock about how difficult glucose control actually is with a "broken pancreas." It's a struggle every day, even for the world's most conscientious patient.

After three years on shots (I used a NovoPen® Junior insulin pen), I decided I was ready for the leap into pumping. But not with tubing, please! I lobbied the folks at Insulet Corporation to set me up with their OmniPod™ tubeless pumping system, even though it wasn't yet commercially available on the West Coast. I have been a loyal user ever since. Meanwhile, I have a bookcase full of glucose meters, diabetes books, carry cases and other paraphernalia that have been sent to my blog for evaluation.

So yes, I've received a lot of free stuff. But rest assured that running a daily Web log is like running any other daily publication: it's time-consuming, hard work. I can't begin to count how many evenings or weekends my husband or one of my kids has shouted up the stairs: "Are you coming down now? Still blogging?!"

As for my daily routine? Like most working moms, I have to be ultra-efficient. Never a minute is wasted. Most weekdays, I get up shortly after 6:00 AM and test my sugar, then prepare breakfast, start a load of wash, feed the cat, pack some lunches, check my Website, make a shopping list, and help my girls get ready before packing them all in the car for our multi-school drop-off. Somewhere in between all that I've got to dose insulin and eat, otherwise I 'm grumpy and useless. After all that, my regular work day begins.

Fitting in workouts is a very high priority. I belong to two different gyms near my home, and I like to jog and take long bike rides when weather and time permit. I have become fairly adept at using my pump's temporary basal settings to cut back on background insulin while working out. But hey, it's a work in progress, like everything else with diabetes. Occasionally I have unpleasant lows that interfere with my workouts, and nothing makes me madder!

Being allergic to wheat makes food choices far trickier than the diabetes alone would do. At home, it's pretty easy to cook with gluten-free ingredients, but restaurants seem to douse everything in flour. I often bring along my own store of gluten-free crackers, especially in case the service is slow and I start to feel shaky with hunger.

When possible, I like to do menu planning on Sunday nights so I can buy the ingredients for several dinners for the coming week in a one-stop-shop. That sure makes my life as a working mom easier.

And speaking of "*schlepping*," I keep a "go-bag" in my car full of diabetes back-ups: an extra meter and batteries, extra pump supplies and insulin, glucose tablets, an extra lancing device, alcohol wipes – you name it! I have learned the hard way that "Murphy's Law" applies all-too-well to diabetes, and you do not want to have to make an emergency trip home every time some little thing inevitably goes wrong.

I've been blessed with a life partner who's my best friend, who's known me long before the diabetes, and has grown into this new life right alongside me. He's a problem-solver of the highest order and an eternal optimist – two golden characteristics when dealing with chronic illness.

Since diving into the diabetes world, I've had the opportunity to meet the most amazing people! Many are "ordinary patients" like me, who manage to cope with the challenges of this illness with courage and grace. They've opened their hearts both online and offline to those who share their plight.

In my role as a diabetes journalist, I've also had the opportunity to interview some of the most famous people touched by diabetes, including singers Nick Jonas, Crystal Bowersox, Angie Stone, and George Canyon; actresses Delta Burke, Olympia Dukakis (whose husband has type 2) and Aida Turturro of "The Sopranos;" Olympic athletes Gary Hall, Jr., and Kris Freeman; rising tennis star Elizabeth Profit; prima ballerina Zippora Karz; global pilot Douglas Cairns; *Amazing Race* winner Dr. Nat Strand; and financier and author Arthur Ainsberg. Hearing about their determination to follow – and conquer! – their dreams despite diabetes has been hugely motivational for me personally: there really are no limits with this illness, as long as you don't allow limitations to be part of your mindset.

Most importantly, this work has made me feel that I am part of something bigger than myself, something truly consequential. I'm constantly in touch with people who are 1) struggling to survive with diabetes, and 2) just as moved by the efforts of fellow PWDs as I am. At DiabetesMine.com, on almost a daily basis, we get e-mails asking questions, sharing personal stories, and/or thanking us for the work we do "connecting the dots" among patients, providers, and diabetes companies. It's more satisfying than any other job I have ever had, and I honestly can't imagine my life now without the online diabetes community. I would be so isolated!

So has diabetes brought some good things into my life? Most certainly. I do believe I live a much more conscious, grateful, and healthful life now than I did before the diabetes, when "health" was taken for granted just like having ten toes. I can certainly relate when people talk about diabetes being "a blessing in disguise." But to my mind, that's only possible *if,* when diabetes alters your life course, you *don't* let it steer you astray. Instead, reach out and grab the steering wheel!

Website: www.DiabetesMine.com
Website: www.DiabeticConnect.com

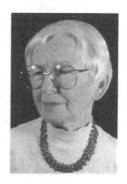

Chapter 24 *by Heartha Whitlow*

My 70-Year Journey with Type 1 Diabetes

Introduction

I grew up in San Antonio, Texas, and considered myself the healthiest person in the world. But I did have one problem: I had an inherited form of rickets and had to wear braces on my legs for many years. I remember how the kids, especially one boy, made fun of me, calling me "Bowlegs." One day I came home crying and told my mother about this. To my complete surprise, she said, "Oh, that poor boy. You must feel sorry for him because he is so ignorant." So, my mother gave me some ammunition that served me well. She was a wonderful, understanding person, and my dad was also a great person.

I was a good student, and my parents wanted me to go to college. But I finished high school at sixteen years old, in 1935, the middle of the Great Depression. My dad, an auto mechanic, had lost his job a long time before, and we subsisted on the money my parents made together by running a hand laundry. So I spent my afternoons helping with the ironing, doing housework, completing my homework, and selling vegetables from our small garden. However, I was encouraged to participate in the interscholastic sports program that Texas schools had at that time. My parents always came to the games against other schools.

Since I was a co-Valedictorian of my high school, I had a scholarship for four years of college. Despite my mother, who urged me to become a teacher, I majored in chemistry.

The Challenge of the Great Depression

When I finished high school, I saw that my family did not have enough money to send me to college; it was mostly up to me to find a way to fund it. I had studied typing in high school, and decided that I needed to study shorthand as well. So I went to a local business college and said, "I need to learn shorthand, but I don't have any money for tuition."

The manager said, "That's okay; we know how things are now. You can take our shorthand course. It will cost $50, and you can pay us later when you get a job." I remember how very proud I was, years later, when I took $50 to the business college to pay for that course.

My first year in college had to be local, so I spent 1935 at Westmoorland College in San Antonio. This was a good experience for me, because a great many things happened. I got a job typing a doctoral thesis for Mrs. Jackson, the wife of the college President, and I earned twenty-five cents a page. I also had a job as secretary to the football coach. I played on the girls basketball team (I was five feet tall), was a member of a poetry club, I worked at the school paper as Sports Editor, and I supplied crossword puzzles in French.

But that year, I also got the mumps. This is significant because about four or five years later. I was diagnosed with type 1 diabetes. At the time, my doctor thought the mumps may have caused my diabetes, because no one else in my family had ever had diabetes. (Currently, researchers are studying the possibility that viral infections can trigger type 1 diabetes in genetically susceptible individuals. There is research that suggests that a viral infection – including mumps – can trigger the onset of type 1 diabetes.)

The next year, 1936, I transferred to the University of Texas at Austin (now called UT Austin), as the university had a very fine reputation. I wanted my chemistry degree to lead to a good job later. Again, the partial tuition scholarship (about $50 as I remember) represented only a small fraction of my total costs. I lived in the least-expensive dormitory, but I still had to buy some very expensive textbooks. My parents paid about half of those costs and I got a job in the chemistry department, earning thirteen cents an hour, to pay for the remaining costs. This was a part of the National Youth Administration (NYA), one of President Roosevelt's attempts to get us through the Depression.

A little later I got a job as secretary to Anna Hiss, Director of Women's Physical Education. My association with her was one of the finest experiences of my life.

During my senior year at UT Austin, my physical chemistry lab instructor was a wonderful guy named Gene Whitlow. We began dating. I graduated with a Bachelor of Science in Chemistry and Phi Beta Kappa from the UT Austin in 1939. Gene and I were married on Christmas Day in 1940.

248

At that time, I was offered a full-time job as the secretary in the Chemistry Department, so my plans for graduate school became somewhat side-tracked. They did allow me to take one graduate course in the department. But there was a nepotism rule, so when we married we had to decide – which one of us could continue working in the Chemistry Department, and who could go for the PhD? I told Gene that I wanted two children and that I would be better equipped to do that job! So, I kept my job, and Gene got a temporary job in the Engineering Department.

The Challenge of Diabetes

In April, Gene suggested that we ought to get insurance policies, and that's when it all began. My physical exam revealed high blood sugar. Since I was a student in graduate school, I went to the physician at the University. She said to me, "I don't know anything about diabetes, but I'll consult with my colleagues in Austin. Since you are a chemist, I think you should take care of this thing yourself." She put me on a long-acting insulin to begin with, and taught me how to inject it.

The injections never bothered me, but my ego took a beating. I remember thinking, *Why me?* Then I said to Gene, "We ought to get a divorce right now. You don't deserve the kind of life we're in for."

Gene replied, "We can handle it."

And then I thought, *Why* not *me?* (I have found that the most helpful thing you can do to adapt is to have a matter-of-fact attitude.) And so, we decided that my diabetes diagnosis would be an interesting challenge for a couple of chemists. Our positive attitude made all the difference.

Gene was completely supportive, but those early years were rough on him. You see, in those days, we couldn't run blood sugar tests. I was given a little kit for checking sugar in my urine. It consisted of a small test tube, a blue tablet (a copper compound), and another tablet which could be set on fire under the tubing. A positive test, which indicated sugar in the urine, would turn the urine orange or red. This was not very accurate, because it gave no indication until sugar was spilled (which I think happened at about 180 mg/dL).

So my attempts at a proper diet were constantly challenged. I remember once when we went to a fancy dinner at which pecan pie was served. I simply took some extra insulin and ate my piece of pie. Later, when I ran my test, I again took some extra insulin.

Due to my casual approach, I often had severe insulin reactions in the middle of the night. My convulsions would wake Gene up, and he would rush to the kitchen, bring a glass of orange juice, and try to hold me up while he poured the orange juice down my throat. We ruined a lot of sheets that way! But I am convinced that Gene saved my life at least a dozen times.

249

World War II

In December of 1941, the Japanese attacked Pearl Harbor, and our lives changed. Gene went to the Draft Board and said, "How can I help?"

He was told, "Since you are a chemist, we'd like you to work in the magnesium plant," which wasn't too far from Austin. So Gene spent his days making magnesium, and his evenings working on the research and thesis for his doctorate. I went to the lab with him and spent my time in the glass-blowing lab learning how to shape glass.

In the daytime, I worked as the secretary for the Department of Chemistry, and picked up some extra money by tutoring chemistry students and typing theses for doctoral students. I also helped teach Chemistry I to a group of Chemical Warfare students, as a part of the war effort.

We didn't have much money, but it was a good life and we made a lot of friends. I don't remember that my diabetes made any difference to my quality of life.

After the War

In 1945, Gene stopped making magnesium and he earned his PhD in Physical Chemistry. (His Bachelor of Science and Master of Science degrees were in Chemical Engineering). We left Austin and moved to Evansville, Indiana, to work for Servel, Inc. They were short of chemists, so I also got a job in the lab analyzing lithium bromide, ammonia, and various freons. I made good use of my glassblowing skills, because a lot of the analytical hardware in the engineering lab had to be made by hand.

During those years, I simply did my best with regards to my blood sugar control. It was complicated by a recurrent fever, diagnosed as *thymus fever*, and it made me tired. But a more important plan was developing: I wanted very much to have a child. Gene was doubtful because of my diabetes. He had two reasons for objecting: first, he thought the diabetes would pose a danger to me, and second he thought our children might develop diabetcs. But my doctor backed me up, and I had no trouble becoming pregnant. My doctor said, "By the time your children are grown, diabetes will have been cured." I sure wish he had been right!

I worked in the lab until my sixth month of pregnancy. Our son, Dana, was born on December 28, 1946 as a Caesarian section delivery. Our daughter, Kerry, was born seven years after Dana as a natural delivery. I had two miscarriages during those seven years in between. During my pregnancies, the thymus fever stopped, but resumed later. I continued trying to control my blood sugar by performing frequent tests and making immediate corrections when they were indicated. I believe that the reason I've survived type 1 diabetes for seventy years is because I never allowed a high blood sugar to remain high for very long. Both the children were born in Evansville, where we lived for about twelve years. We moved back to San Antonio (my home town), where Gene was Chairman of the Department of Chemistry and Chemical Engineering Research at the Southwest Research Institute. The job was very stressful for Gene. Three years later, in 1959, when Whirlpool® offered him a job, we decided to make the move to Saint Joseph, Michigan. Gene was quickly promoted to Manager of Chemistry Research. His job was very rewarding and we made lots of friends.

In 1985, after Gene had worked at Whirlpool® for twenty-five years, he switched to a job at Phillips Engineering, Inc. Ben Phillips, the owner of the company, was an old friend from UT Austin; my first job at UT Austin had been with him. A short time after Gene started working with Ben Phillips, I was also hired to do analyses in Ben's chemistry lab; we had come full circle.

We were with Phillips Engineering, Inc. when I began to have more trouble controlling my blood sugar. It was always difficult to control my blood sugar, and the process required many tests every day, with frequent corrections. In 1995, I began to feel very discouraged. I felt that I was going downhill, and I told Gene that I wanted an insulin pump. But the cost was about $6,000 and it was not covered by our insurance plan. Gene said, "If it will help you, we'll get it anyway." My doctor intervened, so our insurance company did help, after all. My health improved a lot after I went on the insulin pump.

It's Been a Good Life

Being a person with diabetes has not kept me from having a good life. Among the nicest things that happened to me were the times my family and I spent on our sailboat. We bought a sloop (a Pearson 26) while the kids were still young. It had four bunks and a tiny, pendulum stove. (A pendulum stove is a big help on a sailboat because it maintains the attached skillet in a horizontal position.) We went out on weekend cruises along the eastern shore of Lake Michigan. When we were planning a cruise, I prepared our meals ahead of time as though for picnics, and took my usual amounts of insulin. Some of our meals were in restaurants, near the harbors where we tied up our boat, so I simply estimated the insulin dose that I would need.

I don't remember having any problems with my blood sugar control, except for one thing: it was difficult to get enough exercise. When we arrived at ports and stayed for a long enough time, then I was able to take walks.

I remember one day when Dana, Gene and I were involved in a small-boat race and the wind was a little too brisk. The boat was leaning over so far that, with Gene at the helm, Dana and I had to lean far over the windward side with our feet tucked under the hiking strap. But the strap broke, and I went overboard. It took Gene quite awhile to get the boat circled back around to

251

where I was floating in my lifejacket. Dana stuck out an oar to me and helped me climb back aboard. The only casualty was the stopwatch I had been wearing.

Gene and I had wonderful kids, and we sure enjoyed each other. One day, we took our boat up the coast to South Haven and found a slip where we could stay overnight. The next morning, the weather was so bad that it wasn't safe to return home, so we were stuck there. Frankly, it was very boring.

Kerry (I think she was about ten years old at the time) announced that she wanted to bake some biscuits. We had none of the ingredients and no oven, but that was no excuse. So, Dana and I rented a couple of bicycles and left the marina in search of a grocery store. We found one and purchased flour, baking powder, salt, margarine, and milk and brought them back to the boat. Kerry mixed up her biscuits and "baked" them, a few at a time, in the tiny skillet that was our only stove. We had the best-smelling boat in that harbor!

I enjoyed eating those fresh biscuits, as I counted the carbohydrates. I knew that a small biscuit might have ten grams of carbohydrate and I could eat twenty-five grams of carbohydrates at each meal. They were delicious!

Awards

Sometime during the 1990s, I realized that I was eligible for the fifty-year awards given by Eli Lilly and Company and by the Joslin Diabetes Center, so I wrote to them to apply. They wrote back that I had to supply a copy of my birth certificate plus affidavits from someone, preferably a doctor, who was aware of when I'd received my first diagnosis of type 1 diabetes.

I found this requirement very difficult to fulfill. First of all, I was born in Lake Charles, Louisiana, at a time when they were not keeping track of births. (I asked an old friend of my family to write a letter on my behalf.) Also, I think I had to include an early school record that recorded my age. And of course, I had long since lost contact with the doctor I had when I was diagnosed.

Fortunately, both companies accepted my husband's letter about his memory of my first diagnosis. Then I received the two medals. The medal from Eli Lilly and Company is silver, on a silver chain, and has a *big* "50" with the word "Years" below the number, and my name engraved on the back. The medal from the Joslin Diabetes Center is bronze and has a figure, which looks like an Olympic runner, with a lit torch in hand. It says, "Triumph for Man and Medicine" on the front, and is engraved with the words, "For 50 Courageous Years with Diabetes" on the back.

1996 was a year full of happenings for us. That summer was the Grand Opening of the Box Factory for the Arts, of which I was one of the original founding members. (I also served as Treasurer until 2007.) So, early one Saturday morning, I took my camera and went to St. Joseph. There, I found a lot of people gathered for a ribbon-cutting ceremony on the front steps of the Box Factory. There was a state senator, the mayor of St. Joseph, and some other notables. It was very impressive.

Thinking the ceremony was finished, I started to leave, when a friend told me there was more inside. We all entered. We went past the first gallery and up to the beginning of the second gallery. Above the second gallery, there was a large beam, which was covered by a huge blanket. I got my camera ready; when the blanket was removed, I saw painted on the beam, "Heartha Whitlow Gallery." I was completely overwhelmed and found it difficult to photograph. I guess that was the best award I have ever received!

Also in 1996, in early December, we got a call from our son Dana, who was working for a computer firm in Beaverton, Oregon. He said he was in the hospital. He had slipped and fallen on his kitchen floor and broken both his legs, just below the hips. It sounded complicated, so Gene and I decided to go out to Oregon to take care of him. Before we left, I asked a friend to submit one of my paintings for the Art Guild's Annual Poster Contest. It was a fundraising event.

When we got to Oregon, we found that Dana had lots of helpful friends. Two of them had built him a ramp so that he could get back into his house while he was in a wheelchair. One of his neighbors took us grocery shopping. Another friend of his took us to a doctor – when Gene and I, along with most of the people of Portland, got sick in a big flu epidemic. On Christmas day, Dana's neighbors brought in Chinese food and helped us celebrate the holiday.

When we returned home soon after New Year's, I learned that my painting had been accepted for the 1997 poster. It was very satisfying to see my artwork published all over town!

My Poetry

During those years, I began to write more poetry. I was originally inspired by a very fine English teacher in high school. Most of my poems were generally philosophical in nature. I was very active at the Box Factory for the Arts when I decided to collect my best poems in a book, which I thought I could assemble on my computer. But Judy Sokolowski, a Box friend, had a better vision for me and she helped me plan a coffee-table style book in which each poem had a painting that illustrated it. Judy arranged to have the book printed by the Litho Tech at Andrews University. The book is an 8 x 10 spiral bound cover, and the front design shows one of my paintings. Judy is listed as the publisher. I decided to donate the proceeds of this book's sales to the Box Factory, and Judy was able to obtain a grant which paid for the publication costs. We sold enough of these books during the first year (2002) to pay for all the costs. I have since assembled five more books, on my computer, which show both poems and paintings.

My publications are entitled: *Ramblings of a Renaissance Mind* (2002), *More Ramblings I: Whimsies* (2006), *More Ramblings II: Relationships* (2006), *More Ramblings III: Just thinking* (2006), *More Ramblings IV: Searching* (2006), and *More Ramblings V: Glimmerings* (2009).

I went through my books and found one of my poems, "Which Path to Choose." I am proud that this poem has been chosen as the Epilogue to end *MY SWEET LIFE*, as it immediately follows my story. I also painted an original piece of artwork for the occasion of this book. The poem and painting are combined together; I do hope you will enjoy them.

Family Relations

I have always felt guilty about my diabetes being a nuisance to my family. My husband handled most of the problems, but my kids had to be instructed about how to spot *hypoglycemic* reactions. Eventually, I learned that this was not necessarily a negative thing. I believe that life is made of moments, and my memory has recorded a couple of interesting moments in my journey with diabetes.

One of these is about our daughter, Kerry. When she was eleven years old, we found out that her kidneys were beginning to fail. She finally had a transplant when she was seventeen years old. The intervening years were difficult for her – highly restricted, low-protein diet, intensive treatment for high blood pressure, and fatigue. But she didn't let all this keep her from pursuing a normal life. She was a fine musician, earned a degree in Microbiology and a Master's in Plant Pathology. She married a young biochemist, who is still close to me today.

I remember when Kerry and her husband were home for a visit. I said to her, "Kerry, I know you've had a lot of tough luck, and I admire the fact that you have never complained.

Kerry said, "Well, Mom, I saw how you have handled your diabetes, and I have tried to do the same."

That moment remains a precious memory for me. Our daughter died in 1990 at the age of thirty-seven.

Having a very supportive husband has made all the difference for me to live well with diabetes. Gene and I both became artists and enjoyed many "painting holidays" together. Many of my photos later became the basis for some of my best paintings. We went through a lot together.

There is another moment that I remember fondly. It was evening; Gene and I had finished supper, and we had settled into our favorite chairs, each of us with a book. Suddenly, Gene looked at me and said, "You know, you have given me a good life!"

Surprised, I said, "Even though I've been so much trouble for you?"

He said, "Oh, yes." Gene died on July 26, 2009. The memory of that moment still sustains me when I look at his empty chair. I know that I was lucky to have such a fine partner for sixty-nine years.

My son, Dana, came home from his job at the observatory in Puerto Rico, and stayed with me for a while, taking care of the many difficult tasks that became necessary at the time of Gene's death. We remain close, because we e-mail each other often, and he comes home every year for a visit.

The Nuisance of Chemotherapy

Sometime during 2007, I had a mild heart attack. I recovered very well. Then, just before Christmas in 2007, I fell and broke my right leg, just below the titanium rod that had been installed many years earlier as part of a hip replacement. The surgery was complicated, and it was five months before I could put my full weight on that leg.

I spent four and half weeks in a rehabilitation center, and learned one important thing: those organizations are not equipped to handle diabetes. My pump happened to be out of order and I couldn't replace it until the insurance company decided they could cover it. The staff wouldn't let me take my own insulin or run my own tests. Each nurse had eighteen patients to care for, so the proper timing of my shot was impossible, and I was served the same meals as everyone else. I had to guess at the amounts I could eat. During that period, I had two serious episodes of *hypoglycemia*.

Early in 2008, I was diagnosed with ovarian cancer, and have been receiving chemotherapy treatment ever since. The most important side effect is a few days of very high blood sugar, which requires more blood sugar testing and extra insulin. They can't cure the cancer, but they say they can "keep pushing it back." Another side effect is fatigue and muscle weakness. I've painted only a few landscapes and have written only a few poems since I started these treatments.

But I have a lot of friends who are quick to offer help when I need it. I especially enjoy having dinners out with them. My favorite restaurant serves Italian food; I am able to stay on my diet because pasta has a low *glycemic* index.

What a Difference a Pump Makes

I have worked out a very effective method that I use for managing my blood sugar. My favorite blood glucose meter holds the strips in a drum which is easier for me to manage. (I have osteoarthritis, which makes it difficult for me to handle the individual test strips for many meters.) Each drum holds seventeen

255

test strips. I check my blood sugar about ten to twelve times a day; about three of those tests I run during the night.

My system goes like this: I have a full-size data sheet each day. The top half of the sheet consists of a graph, where I plot the results of each test. If the test result is high, I take the necessary insulin bolus, and record that on my data sheet. With my pump, I can take boluses as small as one-tenth of a unit. If the test result is low, I eat a carefully calculated amount of carbohydrates (a mix of fast and slow) and mark the new blood sugar level with a small "x" on my data sheet. I connect these values to the previous tests for that day. My target blood sugar now is 120 mg/dL.

I studied Richard Bernstein's book, *Diabetes Solutions*, which focuses on achieving normal blood sugar for people with diabetes, by following a low carbohydrate diet and exercise. The book helps me to calibrate my insulin/ carbohydrate ratio. I get a blood sugar rise of 7 mg/dL for each gram of carbohydrate. But I weigh only ninety-seven pounds. Most people get a rise of 5 mg/dL for each gram of carbohydrate.

I make extensive use of the *glycemic* index values and I weigh or measure everything I eat. One important thing: I write down my meal before I eat it; this one thing makes it a lot easier to conform to my low-carbohydrate diet. The glycemic index is very important for my blood sugar control. Because I count carbohydrates, I consult it constantly, and try to use at least one low-*glycemic* food with each meal. For low blood sugar, I have a good supply of carbohydrates, both in my kitchen and my bedroom. And, when I leave the house, I always make sure that my blood sugar is high enough to handle any possible drops for the next few hours.

My latest lab test results (in August, 2011) showed my A1C is 6.2 percent. My doctor says that's very good – considering the cancer and my seventy-year journey with type 1 diabetes!

Epilogue

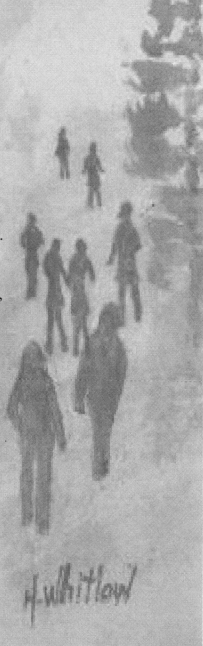

WHICH PATH TO CHOOSE

We are creatures of wishes and yearnings,
Of strivings and hopings that might never be.
But what really counts and what surely matters
Is how do we face all the troubles we see.

You can whine and complain; you can mumble
"Why me?"
Or you can grin and say just, "Why not me?"
And then handle the deal in a matter-of-fact way.

For the truth is—it's part of the human condition,
And luck is a factor in all of our times;
All these upings and downings reveal what
We're made of;
Perhaps they can teach what maturity means?

So—we can choose to be happy,
Or choose to be sad.
But—my life has seen a lot more of the pluses,
So—I choose the path to be grateful—and glad.

Heartha Whitlow
August, 2008

Made in the USA
San Bernardino, CA
27 January 2016